INFORMED CONSENT

INFORMED CONSENT
Legal Theory and Clinical Practice

Paul S. Appelbaum, M.D.
Charles W. Lidz, Ph.D.
Alan Meisel, J.D.

New York   Oxford
OXFORD UNIVERSITY PRESS
1987

Oxford University Press

Oxford New York Toronto
Delhi Bombay Calcutta Madras Karachi
Petaling Jaya Singapore Hong Kong Tokyo
Nairobi Dar es Salaam Cape Town
Melbourne Auckland
and associated companies in
Beirut Berlin Ibadan Nicosia

Published by Oxford University Press, Inc.,
200 Madison Avenue, New York, New York 10016

Oxford is a registered trademark of Oxford University Press

Library of Congress Cataloging-in-Publication Data
Appelbaum, Paul S.
    Informed consent.
    Includes bibliographies and index.
    1. Informed consent (Medical law)—United States.
2. Medical ethics—United States. 3. Physician and
patient—United States. I. Lidz, Charles W.
II. Meisel, Alan. III. Title. [DNLM: 1. Decision
Making. 2. Ethics, Medical. 3. Informed Consent—
legislation. W 32.6 A646i]
KF3827.I5A96 1987 344.73′041 86-16179
ISBN 0-19-503841-X 347.30441

10 9 8 7 6 5 4 3 2 1

Printed in the United States of America
on acid-free paper

P.S.A.
To Dede, my wife

C.W.L.
To my parents, Ted and Ruth Lidz

A.M.
To my parents, Stanley and Bebe Meisel

Foreword

As the authors of *Informed Consent: Legal Theory and Clinical Practice* note, in "the clinical setting, the principles of good medical care and of informed consent, properly conceived, are not in opposition." The strength of this volume lies in the demonstration, not simple assertion, of this view of informed consent and its relationship to clinical care. More than any other volume available, *Informed Consent: Legal Theory and Clinical Practice* achieves a synthesis for the clinician (and for all others interested in legal and ethical theory) that not only explains the idea of informed consent and its evolution in legal theory, but also demonstrates how informed consent can be achieved in clinical settings in useful ways. Thus, the title of the book is both apt and descriptive.

Appelbaum, Lidz, and Meisel, respectively a psychiatrist, sociologist, and law professor, have been working together as a team for many years, attempting to elucidate informed consent as a legal and ethical doctrine and at the same time, with their colleagues, making systematic empirical and clinical studies of the subject.*

---

*Lidz CW, Meisel A, Zerubavel E, Carter M, Sestak R, Roth LH: *Informed*

This book is informed by empirical and conceptual work that now goes back over a decade.

While this book is of course about informed consent, it is also far more than that; it presents an integrated theory of the doctor-patient relationship that not only grounds informed consent in the ethical ideal of respecting patients (by giving them a meaningful opportunity to choose the type of care they wish) but also retains elements of the doctor-patient relationship that are critical for ensuring that patients' health care needs are met. To this end, important and organizing principles are presented—for example, the authors' delineation of consent as a process, not an event; the idea of mutual monitoring of information disclosure and the consent process by patients and doctors so that each understand the rationales for the others' choices; the authors' distinction, both conceptual and practical, between the goals of informed consent for research versus those of treatment. Each of these ideas is explored in depth.

These principles, once explained, set the framework for the reader. In the latter sections of the book, moving from the theoretical to the practical, the authors offer advice about entering into a doctor-patient relationship, making the ideal of informed consent a reality. Thus with this approach, the reader is prepared for the new situations, consent rules, and procedures that undoubtedly will evolve in the future.

In the transitional period we are now witnessing, with a rapidly changing and often confusing health-care delivery system, it has become essential that a meaningful theory be delineated and ac-

---

Consent: A Study of Decisionmaking in Psychiatry. New York, Guilford, 1984. Lidz CW, Meisel A: Informed consent and the structure of medical care, in President's Commision for the Study of Ethical Problems in Medicine and Biomedical Behavioral Research, *Making Health Care Decisions: The Ethical and Legal Implications of Informed Consent in the Patient-Practitioner Relationship* Vol. 3, *Appendices. Empirical Studies of Informed Consent*. Washington, D.C., U.S. Government Printing Office, 1982. Appelbaum PS, Roth LH: Treatment refusal in medical hospitals, in President's Commission for the Study of Ethical Problems in Medicine and Biomedical Behavioral Research, *Making Health Care Decisions: The Ethical and Legal Implications of Informed Consent in the Patient-Practitioner Relationship* Vol. 3, *Appendices. Empirical Studies of Informed Consent*. Washington, D.C., U.S. Government Printing Office, 1982.

cepted that will ensure that patients become knowledgeable participants in choosing health-care options. In an era when fears of malpractice are growing and societal approval is placed on competition and cost cutting (particularly through the development of bureaucratic structures such as health maintenance organizations or HMOs, preferred provider organizations or PPOs, and other types of prepaid or capitation plans), the possibility is that a patient's choices in the future will be overwhelmed by powerful economic and structural forces. This makes it critical that patients understand their situation and the rules of the doctor-patient relationship, and that genuine informed consent for treatment be obtained for reasons other than to comply with legal or regulatory requirements, or to ensure against liability. To accomplish this, a theory of doctor-patient (or investigator-subject) interaction becomes critical for instructing, even inspiring, all the participants in health-care delivery.

The chances are great that while future patients will be told mechanical details about treatments they will receive, they will potentially understand little else—particularly the ground rules for health care under which they are receiving treatment. Fortunately, because of this book's emphasis on ethics (not only legal rules) and its attention to the realities of care (through clinical discussion and case review), the reader learns not only that it is necessary to obtain consent, but why and what good will come of this—perhaps this book's most important message. *Informed Consent: Legal Theory and Clinical Practice* communicates a structure of values that is generalizable and which, I believe, will help future doctor-patient interactions.

The authors are to be congratulated. This book will, I believe, play a seminal role in the education of future generations of medical students, house officers, and practitioners. Its theoretical underpinnings provide a valuable addition to our understanding of the doctor-patient relationship and I hope it is not too late for its message to be heeded.

Loren H. Roth, M.D., M.P.H.

Preface

Few issues affecting the therapeutic professions are as much discussed and as little understood as informed consent. Most physicians, and other professionals who are affected by the legal requirements for informed consent, recognize that there is some legal obligation to talk with patients and obtain their agreement to proposed treatment. But often their knowledge of the details is a mixture of myth and misunderstanding. Few health-care professionals are aware of the ethical principles underlying the idea of informed consent. Their actual legal obligations are often quite different from what they believe. Most important, few caregivers realize that the requirements of informed consent can be met in a manner that improves, and does not impede, patient care.

As researchers and practitioners concerned with informed consent, we have been acutely aware of how little the doctrine is understood. We have each spent much of the last decade studying informed consent from the perspective of physician, social scientist, and lawyer. When asked by friends and colleagues for a reference that might provide a concise and practical overview of informed consent, embodying the practical knowledge that we and others have obtained from years of observational and empirical studies, we were compelled to confess that no such work existed.

In this volume we have attempted to provide health professionals—including physicians, nurses, dentists, podiatrists, optometrists, psychologists, and social workers, among others—with a comprehensive introduction to the theory and practice of informed consent. Although written with the practitioner in mind, we suspect that this book will serve equally well the students, researchers, and attorneys who want to learn more about the development of informed consent law and the problems faced when ethical and legal theories confront the realities of clinical practice.

Part I provides an overview of the development of the idea of informed consent as well as an introduction to the ethical theories on which the idea rests. In Part II, the evolution and current status of the law are described; legal requirements for practitioners are detailed, with particular attention given to areas of legal ambiguity that are problematic for practitioners in formulating their approaches; and the legal theory of informed consent is critiqued.

Part III considers the problems health professionals face when applying informed consent theory in the clinical setting and proposes a model for simplifying that task and making it clinically meaningful. Part IV delineates the unique problems created by the requirements for informed consent in the research setting, especially the clinical investigations. Part V addresses the long-term need to improve practitioners' performance in meeting the ethical and legal mandates, and suggests a course of action.

Our hope is that this book will illuminate the significance of informed consent in clinical practice and provide a model for practitioners to follow. To the extent that we are able to do so, and to convey the fascination we have felt in exploring the nuances of informed consent, we will have succeeded in our goals.

July 1986

P. S. A.
C. W. L.
A. M.

Acknowledgments

The ideas contained in this book have been incubating in each of us for more that a decade. During that time, we have worked, both together and separately, with a large number of colleagues who have influenced our thinking on informed consent. At this distance, it is almost impossible to sort out the contribution each person has made to our thinking and to thank them appropriately. Clearly, though, they deserve our most profound thanks.

Loren Roth, our friend and colleague, brought us together in the Law and Psychiatry Program at the Western Psychiatric Institute and Clinic, in Pittsburgh. His insights into the legal, ethical, and clinical aspects of informed consent are reflected throughout this book in more ways than we can possibly enumerate.

We owe a substantial intellectual debt to Jay Katz, who introduced one of us (A.M.) to this field, and whose vision of informed consent has been so influential in both the legal and clinical communities.

Others to whom we are grateful for their intellectual support in studying informed consent include Alexander M. Capron and Egon Bittner. Our colleagues over a number of years in the Law and Psychiatry Program at the University of Pittsburgh also deserve our thanks: Mary Carter, Jeffrey Geller, Anne McHugh, Edward Mulvey, Regina Sestak, Robert Wettstein, and Eviatar Zerubavel.

The empirical studies on which much of our understanding of informed consent is based were funded by the Center for Studies in Crime and Delinquency and Mental Health Services Development Branch, National Institute of Mental Health; the Foundations Fund for Research in Psychiatry; and the President's Commission for the Study of Ethical Problems in Medicine and Biomedical and Behavioral Research. This book is a culmination of these studies in this area.

Many research assistants aided us over the years in collecting information that ultimately appears in this volume. Our thanks to Julie Broido, Ronald Hartman, Robert Hilgendorff, Christopher T. Katucki, Stanley Milavec, Susan Muse, Linda Pingitore, Richard Ruth, Dominic Salvatori, and especially Lisa D. Kabnick and Martha J. Greer. LuAnn Driscoll's untiring and always cheerful efforts as director of the word processing center at the University of Pittsburgh School of Law were most appreciated, as was the secretarial assistance of Sue Wildfeur.

Finally, we acknowledge the most important support of Thomas Detre, for many years the chairman of the Department of Psychiatry, University of Pittsburgh School of Medicine, whose encouragement to explore informed consent and related issues was invaluable. Thanks are due as well to the current chairman, David Kupfer, and the chairman of the Department of Psychiatry, University of Massachusetts Medical School, Aaron Lazare, for their support.

Contents

PART II THE LEGAL THEORY OF INFORMED CONSENT

I

AN INTRODUCTION TO INFORMED CONSENT

1

Informed Consent: Framing the Questions

What is informed consent? The answer may seem self-evident only to those who have yet to explore the many meanings of the term. Informed consent refers to legal rules that prescribe behaviors for physicians in their interactions with patients and provide for penalties, under given circumstances, if physicians deviate from those expectations; to an ethical doctrine, rooted in our society's cherished value of autonomy, that insures to patients their right of self-determination when medical decisions need to be made; and to an interpersonal process whereby physicians (and often other health-care professionals) interact with patients to select an appropriate course of medical care.

Informed consent is each of these things, yet none of them alone. As a theory based on ethical principles, given effect by legal rulings, and implemented by clinicians, it has been haunted by its complex lineage. When legal principles and ethical values conflict, which should take precedence? When clinical interests appear to be served by neither legal nor ethical concerns, which interests should be compromised and to what degree? The vast literature on informed consent, found in journals and books of medicine, law, philosophy, and public policy, has been stimulated by the need to create a workable doctrine that can accommodate values that to many observers are in an irremediable state of conflict.

The conflicts in theory and the need to resolve them in practice are the subjects of this book. Theory is the focus of the first half of the volume; practice is the topic of the second. Seeking to understand the fascinating theoretical problems requires us to grapple with some of the most difficult ethical and policy issues facing our society today. But let us state at the outset our belief that the clinician on the front lines need not be paralyzed by differences of opinion between legal and ethical theorists. Through the vaguely translucent wall of expertise behind which the discussion about the proper shape of the informed consent doctrine has taken place, a reasonable approach to informed consent in the clinician-patient relationship can be discerned. Our most important and challenging task in this book is to make that approach evident.

Since the goal of this volume is to help the clinician deal reasonably with legal and ethical mandates for informed consent, we begin our analysis in the clinical setting. From a consideration of informed consent in practice emerge the questions we address in the rest of this book.

1.1 The Clinical Setting

John Williamson (all names have been altered in this history of an actual case) is a 23-year-old man who was seen in an outpatient surgical clinic of a major health center and diagnosed as suffering from an acute flare-up of chronic pancreatitis. Mr. Williamson's chief complaint was the intense abdominal pain that accompanies pancreatitis. Dr. Johnson, the chief surgical resident, had seen him a number of times before for similar problems. Dr. Johnson and Dr. Ricah, the senior resident, examined him and asked whether the narcotic pain relievers they had previously prescribed were doing him any good.

> Patient: No. . . . I am just getting used to them. Maybe a couple of belts (i.e., drinks) would help me out.
>
> Chief Resident: No, I can guarantee that that will not help. . . . I've

looked at your tests but I still want to look at your X-rays. What I think is that you will do better if we take out part of your pancreas; as long as you understand that this is a serious operation in that, while you probably won't die from it, there is a small chance that you might, although not much. But there are serious side effects from it, like you will probably have some diabetes and have trouble digesting your food. Then I think that we should go ahead and have you talk with your wife about coming in and make plans for you to come in.

Senior Resident: I think that you ought to understand that this is not going to be a cure-all. This is not going to do away with all of your problems. You are still going to have a lot of problems from that pancreas of yours.

Patient: I know that.

A researcher studying informed consent, who made daily rounds with the surgical team, witnessed the above conversation and later that morning interviewed Mr. Williamson.

Researcher: Can you tell me what your problem is?

Patient: It is the pancreas.

Researcher: Have any idea why?

Patient: No, I don't know. The doctor knows really what I'll have to do. . . . I've been having this problem about two years now. It's getting unbearable. Before, I could live with it, but now I'll take a chance on anything. . . .

Researcher: Can you tell me what they are going to do in this operation?

Patient: They are going to take my pancreas out.

Researcher: The whole pancreas?

Patient: Um-hm. . . . It is going bad anyway. I'd rather have it out of me than if it really might ruin me on the inside. . . .

Researcher: Think it will make the pain better?

Patient: Well, at least we won't take any chances.

Mr. Williamson was brought into the hospital one week later, after he complained that he was unable to wait the scheduled month before the operation because of the pain. Dr. Johnson described the case on rounds as being one in which he had treated the patient with painkillers for an extensive period of time. He described Mr. Williamson as an ex-alcoholic whose pancreatic deterioration was the result of alcoholism. Dr. Johnson said that he would not make a final decision about going through with the operation until he saw whether or not the X-rays showed that the lesion was limited to an operable area of the pancreas. In his view, the main advantage of the operation was that it would allow Mr. Williamson to be withdrawn from the pain medication. He also said he hoped the patient was telling the truth when he said he had quit drinking, or he would just have the same problem again.

The next day Dr. Johnson revealed to the surgical team on rounds that he planned to do a distal pancreatectomy. "That should benefit him if he has really quit drinking. . . . He has said that he wants it out. The results are not good with distal pancreatectomies but it is probably worth a try. . . . He knows we are doing it to get him off medication." The next morning Dr. Ricah told Mr. Williamson that the X-ray had come back and that they planned to do the operation the next week.

While waiting in the hospital for the tests to be completed and for the scheduled surgery, Mr. Williamson generally was told a little bit about what was happening each day. Four days before the scheduled operation, Dr. Johnson told him, "I'd say that there is a 50 percent chance that there will be no pain after the operation and an 80 to 90 percent chance that it will help you. The object is to relieve some of your pain, and as far as that is concerned the only other thing that we're concerned with is that you've got to be sure you don't drink, because that's not helping at all. So we are going ahead Wednesday, O.K.?" Mr. Williamson agreed.

The next day Mr. Williamson asked about his sugar test. The surgeon responded, "Your sugar seems to be normal. I think if we only have to take out half or two-thirds of the pancreas that you should not become diabetic. You may have to watch your diet a little bit, but that is all." In another interview that afternoon it became clear that Mr. Williamson now understood that only part of the pancreas would be removed, but his description seemed to imply that it was being removed to prevent the spread of an infection.

Two days before the operation, during rounds, the following discussion occurred:

Patient:	How long will the operation take?
Senior Resident:	Four or five hours. It's a pretty long one. I want you to know that we may have to take out your spleen as well as your pancreas.
Patient:	What is that?
Senior Resident:	Oh, it's an organ that takes care of things like the breakdown of old blood cells and a few things like that. It seems to have something to do with fighting infections, so for people who have it taken out, we usually make a special effort to vaccinate them again. We will try to save it, but the blood vessels that feed it run right along the back of the pancreas and it is much better to take it out than to get all of the bleeding that is sometimes required to save the blood vessels. . . . Another problem we could have is adhesions.
Patient:	What's that?
Senior Resident:	Well, because you have had this many operations, things get sticky in there, and we may have trouble with things getting stuck together.
Patient:	What about the diabetes thing?
Senior Resident:	The chances are that you will not have to take any medicine but you may have to watch your diet a bit.

Although Dr. Johnson was convinced that this operation was a good idea, his senior resident was not, and they argued about it more than once. Dr. Ricah felt the patient was expecting too much from the treatment and it was not going to provide him with the relief he expected. Dr. Johnson contended, "There are risks, but I've explained them to him and I'll explain them to him again tomorrow. I think we can help this kid."

The afternoon before the operation Dr. Johnson did the informed consent disclosure required of him by hospital rules.

Chief Resident:	We've talked about everything, I think. We're going to take out that area of the pancreas that is abnormal, and we will probably also have to take out your spleen as

well. The problems of the operation are the possibility of bleeding during the operation. Sometimes there is a possibility of infection from the operation. We will cover you with antibiotics, of course, both before and after the operation. When you come out of the operation you'll have a drain in your nose and in your stomach for a few days. It isn't an easy operation but I am fairly confident that we can help you.

Later that evening one of the evening shift nurses went into Mr. Williamson's room to get a consent form signed.

Nurse: John, I have to get your consent, but you did talk to Dr. Johnson about it today, didn't you?

Patient: (nods)

Nurse: First let me tell you what will happen tomorrow. As soon as we're through here, I am going to start an IV on you and then you're going to get a PhisoHex shower; you know that, don't you?

Patient: (nods)

Nurse: (Describes morning shower, blood pressure monitoring, Valium administration, and starting general anesthesia. Reports that the operation will take four or five hours and tells the patient that he will then come back up to the ward and describes some of the postoperative care. About 10 minutes of description.) Well, all I have left is for you to sign this [consent form]. Read it over first. If you have any questions, just ask. (She leaves the room briefly while he reads a general consent form for surgical procedures containing information specific to his situation.)

Patient: Sign here right? (signing)

Nurse: Do you have any questions?

Patient: Not really. (after a moment) I do have one question. Does my spleen have anything to do with my having children?

Nurse: (surprised) No, no, nothing to do with that.

Mr. Williamson had his operation the next morning.

Mr. Williamson's case is in some ways typical of and in some ways quite different from most doctor-patient interactions. The ambiguities in communication and the unspoken motives of all participants is, current research suggests, common to the medical setting. On the other hand, despite important omissions and Mr. Williamson's less-than-perfect understanding of the reasons for and possible consequences of the procedure he was to undergo, quite a bit of information was passed to Mr. Williamson by his physicians. Existing empirical research, as we shall see, indicates that this is not universally the case.

For our purposes, any conclusions we might draw from interaction between these physicians and their somewhat bewildered patient are of much less importance than the questions raised.

1. The discussions Drs. Johnson and Ricah had with their patient, culminating in his encounter with the nurse who brought him a consent form for his signature, are a part of the preoperative routine (some might say ritual) in most medical centers. Asked why they were doing what they did, most of the participants would probably have replied, "I am trying to live up to my responsibilities under the law of informed consent." What is the law of informed consent and how did it evolve into its current form?

2. Had Dr. Johnson been asked whether he would have behaved differently in the absence of a legal requirement for him to discuss certain issues with his patient, he might well have hesitated before responding. "I'm not sure," he might have replied, "because I've just taken for granted that this is something that we have to do. But now that I think about it, I'd feel uncomfortable operating on someone without telling him something about the operation. It's his body, after all. And besides, he'll be more cooperative if he knows what's going on." This response suggests that the conveyance of information from doctor to patient has roots that go deeper than the legal rules that usually dominate most discussions of consent. Basic notions of right and wrong and good and bad seem to be involved. What are the ethical underpinnings of consent in the doctor-patient relationship?

3. Although Drs. Johnson and Ricah may have felt both legal and ethical imperatives to provide Mr. Williamson with certain information concerning his medical care, they were clearly selective. Mr. Williamson was told some of the major risks of surgery, for example, but never that his physicians viewed the operation largely as a maneuver to wean him from the use of painkillers or that they had substantial doubts that the procedure would mea-

surably reduce his pain. There was no discussion at all of possible alternatives to the distal pancreatectomy Dr. Johnson decided to perform. What information does the law require physicians to disclose to their patients when it defines what constitutes an informed consent?

4.   Mr. Williamson, who had barely completed high school, had obvious difficulty understanding some of the information his physicians communicated to him. In part, this problem may have resulted from the lack of detail he was offered. The discussion of diabetes as a possible consequence of the surgery, for example, was conducted without any effort to explain to Mr. Williamson just what it might mean to cope with a surgically induced diabetic state. But some of Mr. Williamson's confusion stemmed from his own intellectual limitations. Was he able to understand enough of what he was told to make a meaningful decision about surgery? How can one determine who is able to make their own decisions—in legal terms, who is competent to decide for themselves—and who is not? When someone is found not to be competent, what alternative decisionmaking mechanisms are available?

5.   Lurking in the back of the minds of the physicians in this case was the knowledge that some doctors are subjected to suit by their patients on the grounds that informed consent was not obtained. On what basis can such suits be brought and according to what rules are they handled by the legal system?

6.   The procedure Dr. Johnson performed on Mr. Williamson is an accepted part of the surgical repertoire, not an innovation that Dr. Johnson decided to test. Furthermore, Dr. Johnson's sole motivation for performing the surgery was to help Mr. Williamson, rather than in a formal way to gather data that might be of assistance to other patients in the future. What if the opposite had been the case? That is, what if Dr. Johnson had been introducing a new surgical procedure and intended to use information about Mr. Williamson's operation as part of a larger body of data to assess the new procedure's utility? Would the ethical or legal rules governing consent change? Should consent be obtained differently in such circumstances?

The questions stated so far address primarily the theoretical aspects of informed consent from an ethical and legal perspective.

Mr. Williamson's case also raises a number of practical questions concerning informed consent in the clinical setting.

7. As we have seen, questions exist about how effective the efforts to communicate with this patient really were, and how much he was able to comprehend, regardless of the communication methods used. What do we know about various methods of disclosure? How much do patients understand as a result? How competent are most patients? Finally, how are decisions about medical care really made?

8. Careful review of the transcripts of Mr. Williamson's discussions with his caregivers suggests some puzzling and troubling issues. For example, Mr. Williamson was given a good deal of information about his treatment over a period of several days. However, he appears to have committed himself to proceed with the surgery well before all the information about it was made available, even before its full extent and major complications were made known to him. (He was unaware that a splenectomy would be part of the procedure until quite late in the process.) What suggestions can we make to Drs. Johnson and Ricah as to how they might better have dealt with Mr. Williamson to ensure a more informed decision?

9. One of the more curious aspects of the interactions was the late appearance on the scene of a nurse bearing a consent form for Mr. Williamson to sign. What purpose do these consent forms have, and are there ways of using them that integrate them more meaningfully into the rest of the informing process?

10. Mr. Williamson consented to have the procedure performed even though he evidently had some serious concerns about the possible results. He signed the consent form, after all, while still entertaining the possibility that the removal of his spleen might have an adverse impact on his ability to father children. What if he had refused to undergo the procedure? Do we have any understanding of why patients refuse treatment, what role the provision of information to them plays in their refusal, and how refusals might best be responded to?

11. A great deal of ink has been spilled in efforts to determine how Mr. Williamson and his doctors should interact before his consent to surgery is considered legitimate. How would critics of

the present process have altered the discussions? Are legal approaches the best way to go about modifying the behavior of both sides?

These general issues, of immense significance for the delivery and receiving of medical care today, and many more related questions, form the substance of the chapters that follow.

1.2 Terminology

Informed consent is a term that has been elaborated in the context of ethics, law, and medicine. As a consequence, the term may denote quite different things to specialists in different disciplines, even at the most general level and among persons to whom informed consent is not a novelty. For example, the phrase *theory of informed consent* may signify one thing to the ethicist and a quite different thing to a person trained in law. Even within a given discipline there may be disparities of understanding as to the meaning of particular terms. The phrase *law of informed consent* may mean one thing to the legal scholar and something else to the trial attorney. As a result, it is necessary to describe here some terms and concepts that appear in discussions of informed consent and to indicate how we will employ them.

The Idea of Informed Consent

At the most general theoretical level is what we call, borrowing from Jay Katz, "the idea of informed consent" (1,p.xvi). *This idea is the core notion that decisions about the medical care a person will receive, if any, are to be made in a collaborative manner between patient and physician.* The concept also implies that the physician must be prepared to engage in—indeed to initiate—a discussion with the patient about the available therapeutic options and to provide relevant information on them. The influential report on informed consent of the President's Commission for the Study of Ethical Problems in Medicine was premised on the *idea* of informed consent, and the report's recommendations strongly reflect the associated concepts (2).

The idea of informed consent has its origins in law, in ethics, and in contemporary understanding in medicine itself about the nature of the doctor-patient relationship and the advantages that accrue when patients are knowledgeable about their treatment. There are two major theories of ethics in the Western tradition. Deontological ethics derive from intrinsic notions of good and bad, and consequentialist ethics are based on the desirability of the results of a policy or action. Both have been applied in the development of the idea of informed consent. (These theories as they relate to informed consent are discussed in Chapter 2.)

Law has also played an important role in nourishing the idea of informed consent. In fact, it is probably from law that the term informed consent originated. Legally protected interests—primarily bodily integrity and individual autonomy—have contributed to the idea of informed consent. The right of bodily integrity is largely a common-law one, embodied in the protections conferred by both the civil and criminal law of assault and battery. There are also important constitutional underpinnings to this right. Individual autonomy, or the right to choose or decide, has similar common-law and constitutional antecedents.

The Legal Doctrine

The idea of informed consent is made operational by means of the *legal doctrine of informed consent.* The doctrine, which prevails in all American jurisdictions with the possible exception of Georgia (3), requires that informed consent be obtained before a physician is legally entitled to administer treatment to a patient. This requirement is actually composed of two separate but related legal duties imposed on physicians: the duty first to disclose information to patients, and the duty subsequently to obtain their consent before administering treatment. (The legal doctrine of informed consent is discussed in Chapters 3 through 6.)

The extent to which the idea of informed consent is actually embodied in legal requirements has been a matter of great concern to scholarly commentators. In practice the idea of informed consent and its ethical and legal underpinnings have been seriously diluted in the duties the law actually imposes on physicians. A similar dilution has been seen in the "rules for recovery" (see below) that govern lawsuits brought by patients who allege that they were treated without informed consent, by which they usually mean that they believe the treatment was inadequately explained to them before they received it.

The *legal requirements for informed consent* generally specify what kind of information doctors must disclose to patients and sometimes how consent should be obtained. An example of these legal requirements is the generally accepted rule that physicians must inform patients of the nature, purpose, risks, and benefits of any treatment they propose to perform, as well as any alternative forms of treatment that may exist for the patients' conditions. Similarly, the exceptions that exist for either making such disclosure or obtaining consent, or both, are also examples of what we mean by the phrase *legal requirements for informed consent*. The legal requirements and levels of specificity vary substantially from state to state and sometimes even from case to case within a given state. It is certainly safe to say that there is no single set of legal requirements for informed consent.

The Rules for Recovery

The legal requirements for obtaining informed consent define the legal obligations of physicians to their patients. The enforcement of these obligations requires further discussion. There are any number of potential means for implementing the idea of informed consent. One might be through requirements promulgated by hospitals, with penalties such as curtailment or loss of staff privileges for the physician who fails to comply. Similarly, in some jurisdictions, such failure may be grounds for state disciplinary proceedings.

By far the most familiar, however, and probably the most common means of redress for a patient who claims there was inadequate explanation and consent prior to treatment, is a lawsuit seeking damages (i.e., a monetary recovery) from the physician. Most such lawsuits are resolved either through settlement procedures or by a trial. Of those that go to trial, a small proportion are appealed. The appellate court reviews the outcome of a trial, determines whether it should be affirmed or reversed, and—most important for present purposes—writes an opinion explaining its reasons for affirmance or reversal. It is from the collected opinions

of appellate courts that the legal requirements for informed consent
are derived, and from which the legal *doctrine* of informed consent
has been developed by scholars, as an embodiment of the *idea* of
informed consent.

Because the opinions are written in response to particular claims
by injured patients requesting compensation for their injuries, the
cases establish a variety of rules to guide the litigation process in
such lawsuits. We refer to these as the *rules for recovery*, that is,
recovery by the patient of damages. Some of these rules involve
the standard of care, the standard of causation, the requirement
for expert testimony, and the materialized risk requirement. These
are largely technical issues, most of which should have only indirect
(though not necessarily insubstantial) effect on the manner in
which physicians seek to comply with their duties to inform patients
and obtain their consent. They deal, in effect, not with the right
to informed consent, but with the remedy for the violation of that
right. (These rules are discussed in Chapter 6.)

The Participants in Decision Making

Finally, let us clarify how providers and recipients of care are
referred to in this volume. Although the legal theory and requirements concerning informed consent have developed almost entirely
in the medical context, psychologists, nurses, social workers, podiatrists, optometrists, physical therapists, chiropractors, and other
professionals who offer treatment to persons who seek their assistance are all affected by and need to know about the theory and
practice of informed consent. For historical reasons, for the sake
of simplicity, and because the physician-patient relationship is still
the most common locus for the application of informed consent,
we refer to caregivers as physicians or doctors in this book. These
terms should be understood to include caregivers of all professions
who are involved in consent situations.

Some of the health-care professionals who are concerned with
the application of the idea of informed consent may use the word
client, or some other term, to refer to the people they serve. Just
as we have chosen physicians as the modal caregivers, we shall
refer to those who receive treatment as patients. The only exception to both these rules comes in discussion of the research setting,

when the terms researcher (or investigator) and subject will be used.

References

1. Katz J: *The Silent World of Doctor and Patient*, New York, Free Press, 1984.

2. President's Commission for the Study of Ethical Problems in Medicine and Biomedical and Behavioral Research: *Making Health Care Decisions: The Ethical and Legal Implications of Informed Consent in the Patient-Practitioner Relationship.* Vol. 1, *Report.* Washington, D.C., U.S. Government Printing Office, 1982.

3. Young v. Yarn, 222 S.E.2d 113 (Ga. 1975).

2

Underlying Ethical Principles

When Dr. Johnson and Mr. Williamson discussed the proposed pancreatectomy in the case described in the previous chapter, were their behaviors affected primarily by ethics or by law? Many of the ethical theories used to justify the idea of informed consent have their roots in beliefs that have animated American society since its founding and can be traced far back in our Judeo-Christian heritage. In this sense, it might be argued that the influence of ethics has been primary. On the other hand, the courts took the initiative in creating the law of informed consent, drawing on equally ancient legal principles. Much of the ethical justification for the law of informed consent has been applied in a post hoc manner. In that sense, the law's influence has been predominant.

The dispute for primacy between law and ethics is ultimately a sterile one. A more useful approach acknowledges that both traditions have contributed to the evolution of informed consent, interacting with each other in a complex manner. Legal initiatives have influenced the development of ethical theories, and they in turn have further stimulated the development of the law. To understand informed consent, therefore, one must consider both its legal and ethical dimensions. This chapter addresses the latter.

2.1 Theories of Ethics

A variety of theories command the attention of medical ethicists. However, there are two dominant trends of thought: deontological ethics and consequentialist ethics, the most important form of which is utilitarian ethics. Both seem almost obvious on first acquaintance, but on closer viewing many difficulties and contradictions emerge.* Both theories can be, and frequently are, used to justify and explicate the duties involved in informed consent.

Deontological Ethics

The word deontological comes from the Greek *deon*, meaning "duty" or "binding." The core of deontological ethics is the identification and justification of duties that are both binding for an individual and more or less independent of the practical concerns facing that individual. Deontologists believe there are ethical obligations that must be fulfilled even if the consequences of fulfilling them are unfortunate. Although many deontological thinkers buttress their ethical arguments by trying to show the practical benefits that will result from fulfilling one's obligations, they see a duty as existing independent of its practical outcome.

Deontological ethics undoubtedly originate in religion. For example, the Ten Commandments lay down ethical obligations that are founded in the Divine Word. When Moses brought the Israelites the commandment *Thou shalt not covet thy neighbor's house*, he did not suggest that it would lead to more peaceful intergroup relations or better mental health. It was enough that God had so commanded. One of the traditional functions of religions is to provide an unassailable foundation for ethical injunctions and legal structures. In the eighteenth century Immanuel Kant revolutionized deontological ethics by developing a secular grounding for ethical duties. This grounding still influences our ethical debates.

Kant's central idea was that the evaluation of any ethical duty requires an assessment of whether it is consistent with a general

---

*An excellent review of deontological and consequentialist theories of ethics is contained in Tom Beauchamp and James Childress, *Principles of Biomedical Ethics*, 2nd edition, New York: Oxford University Press, 1983.

rule he called the categorical imperative. He provided several different expressions of the categorical imperative, but in general it can be taken to mean that one should "act only on a maxim by which you can will that it, at the same time, should become a general law" (1, p.473). In other words, the test of whether a rule should be treated as an ethical duty is whether one can insist that everyone else (or at least everyone who holds a similar position, e.g., all physicians) behave in the same fashion.

Kant believed every moral duty could be assessed in this manner. For example, he sought to show that it was impossible to lie ethically. If one asserts that it is good to lie, one unavoidably raises the question of whether the statement is itself a lie and therefore false. Thus, the universalization of the principle of lying leads to self-contradiction. Similarly, Kant believed that he could derive from the categorical imperative the idea that one must always treat another human being as an end and never merely as a means to another end. This approach to ethics, which clearly places respect for the individual as one of the highest principles, is the part of Kantian ethics that most frequently is cited to justify the idea of informed consent.

Kantian ethics, despite its admirable generality and clarity, has not been without its critics. He seems to provide a wonderfully general rule, but it is not entirely clear that it can be used to assess, in a consistent manner, situations where two principles conflict. For example, how does one assess the ethics of giving distorted information to patients who must decide on their treatment and whom one fears will refuse life-saving therapy if the real information is disclosed? There is a conflict here of two ethical duties: the duty not to lie, and the duty to seek to do good for others. Kantian ethics do not resolve this clash.

Consequentialist Ethics

The consequentialists hold that the rightness or wrongness of an act is dependent on the consequences of the act. This idea may sound suspiciously like the position that the end justifies the means, but it is not the same. Consequentialist positions are the basis of much current political and ethical thinking that sets very high standards for conduct.

The dominant form of consequentialist ethics has been utilitarianism, a position developed by Jeremy Bentham and John Stuart Mill in the early nineteenth century (2,3). The utilitarians were so named because of their belief that the maximization of utility is the goal of all human action. Bentham identified utility with "pleasure" and Mill identified it with "happiness." For both men these terms certainly had a more general meaning than is usual for us today.

Bentham's basic ethical principle was that one should evaluate alternative possible acts on the basis of which would produce the "greatest good for the greatest number" of people, in other words, the greatest collective utility. At the time of its development, a system of ethics that counted all people as equals irrespective of class, gender, or nationality was seen as quite radical. Some such orientation to the collective good prevents consequentialist theories from degenerating into mere justifications of personal convenience. However, this notion of absolute equality can lead to disturbing consequences in the medical setting, where health-care professionals are generally expected to put duty to patients above abstract consideration of overall societal benefits. Yet if one were to take Bentham further, the patient might be considered just another individual to whom no more or less is due than to a stranger on the street, the sole duty being to maximize the general good. While we might all subscribe to Bentham's maxim in the abstract, we would surely be shocked and outraged if a surgeon refused to provide us with a life-saving appendectomy on the grounds that the several thousands dollars would save more lives if it were used to feed starving children in Africa. Yet, as long as the surgeon's calculation of the costs and benefits was correct, the demands of pure utilitarian ethics would be met. Obviously Bentham's position, like Kant's, can sometimes be problematic.

Bentham's ideas have also come under attack from within the consequentialist position in two different ways. First, many have criticized his identification of utility with pleasure. This sort of hedonism is considered objectionable for a number of reasons, including the fact that for some individuals pleasure is not the primary goal of existence. Many consequentialists have countered that hedonism is not an essential feature of consequentialist theory. Indeed, one may desire to promote ends like knowledge or world peace instead of pleasure or happiness. However, because of the wide variety of possible goals, this position rapidly undercuts the unity of utilitarian theory and produces an almost endless number of different ethical systems. Thus, most utilitarians have moved in the direction of viewing utility as the satisfaction of individual preferences, leaving the specification of what those preferences are completely to the discretion of the individuals involved in the situation.

The second objection to classic Benthamite utilitarianism comes from a group of revisionists who call themselves rule-utilitarians, as distinct from the act-utilitarians, the Benthamite type. As Richard Brandt has put it, "a rule-utilitarian thinks that right actions are the kind permitted by the moral code optimal for the society of which the agent is a member. An optimal code is one designed to maximize welfare or what is good (thus, utility)" (4). The rule-utilitarian believes in rules. The individual is neither expected nor permitted to assess every potential act anew, but must follow some sort of moral code, be it one that society has constructed in accordance with the goal of maximizing utility or a privately constituted utilitarian code. This position moves utilitarianism much closer, at least in appearance, to deontological ethics, because it now accepts rules, and a duty to follow them, as the central component of ethics.

Deontological and consequentialist ethicists will often come to the same conclusion, but not always. Consider the example of the physician who lies to a patient so that the patient will accept a treatment necessary to maintain life. Should such lies be permitted? In most deontological ethics, lies can be shown generally to be a violation of the individual's duty. In simple consequentialist ethics, one must evaluate the rule simply on the basis of its expected consequences, which include in this case the maintenance of a life.

2.2 The Principle of Autonomy

Although deontologists and consequentialists often differ on how best to approach problems, many ethicists from both camps have sought to clarify the underlying principles that ought to guide behavior. Then any action can be considered in the light of what a principled action would look like under the same circumstances. If there were but one ethical principle, as certain moral fundamentalists would have us believe, then ethics might not present such a quandary to human beings. In fact, both professional ethicists and lay people usually recognize that there are a variety of principles to be considered when thinking about whether or not a behavior is good.*

To say that a variety of principles must be recognized in ethics, and medical ethics in particular, is not to say that anything will do. Just as one may argue about whether Bach or Mozart (or even John Lennon) was the greatest composer, there is room for argument about many issues in ethics. On the other hand, just as anyone will agree that Itzak Perlman plays more beautiful music than a 4-year-old violinist at the second lesson, so there is a large area of agreement about what ethical principles are important.

Bioethicists have come to a substantial consensus about basic principles. The Belmont Report of the National Commission for the Protection of Human Subjects of Biomedical and Behavioral Research identifies and articulates four fundamental principles: autonomy, nonmaleficence, beneficence, and justice (5). Informed consent is justified almost exclusively under the principle of autonomy. (Aspects of the principles of nonmaleficence and beneficence, the duties to avoid harming others and to do good for others, which at times may represent competing values, are considered in Section 2.4.)

Autonomy is generally recognized as desirable, both intuitively and in the context of the political and social history of our civilization. When the founders of the United States spoke about liberty, they were referring to a right to be treated by the state as an autonomous human being. When the hippies in the 1960s spoke somewhat less elegantly of "being allowed to do my own thing," they too were calling upon the principle of autonomy to justify their relationship to authority.

The concept of autonomy refers to personal freedom of action,

---

*Pluralistic deontology, first articulated by the English philosopher W. D. Ross earlier in this century, recognizes that a variety of *prima facie* duties (or principles) produce actual obligations in a concrete situation. However, Ross provided no adequate means for reconciling conflicting duties.

or the right to do as one pleases, within certain restrictions. The manner of defining these restrictions differs among ethical theories. The principle of autonomy in general ethics refers to respect for the autonomy of others. In bioethics, the principle of autonomy primarily refers to the obligation of health-care professionals to respect the right of patients to make their own decisions about their treatment—the core of the idea of informed consent.

Autonomy has played an enormous part in the development of Western ethics. In connection with the concepts of liberty and freedom, autonomy has been basic to Western political ethics. In one form or another, almost all deontological justifications of the doctrine of informed consent, and some important utilitarian ones, are derivative of the principle of autonomy.

The Meaning and Ethical Grounding of Autonomy

What is autonomy exactly? A close look at Kant and Mill on autonomy shows they were not talking about precisely the same thing. Central to Kant's thought was the freedom of the individual to pursue the dictates of a self-legislated ethical system. Individual autonomy for Kant was not simply an ethical precept; it was the foundation of his entire philosophy. The individual's effort to reason about that which was experientially presented justified the ethical primacy of the autonomous individual. In Kant's words,

> Rational nature exists as an end in itself. Man necessarily conceives of his own existence as being this rational nature. . . . But every other being regards its existence similarly for the same rational reason that holds true for me. . . . Accordingly, the practical imperative will be as follows: Act so as to treat man, in your own person as well as in that of anyone else, always as an end, never merely as a means (1, pp. 474–475).

The emphasis is on the freedom to do what is right as privately understood.

Mill was less concerned with the individual's internal processes. In his vision, utility would be maximized as long as the individual knew what produced personal happiness and was allowed to act on that knowledge. If the maximization of such individual desires were seen as the main goal of human action, it followed that individuals should be permitted the maximum freedom to pursue their personal happiness, consistent with allowing others that same right. This idea is the core of Mill's famous argument in *On Liberty* (3).

Constraints on Autonomy

There are two general constraints on autonomy. The first arises from the individual's relations with the external world. In order to be able to choose freely, one must not be under too much pressure from the outside. Law has two terms that characterize such pressures: coercion and undue influence. The presence of either invalidates the legal character of any effort at producing autonomous expressions, including the granting of consent. Since almost all actions are to some degree pressured by outside circumstances and/or under the influence of someone else, the difficult question is how much influence or coercion must be present for a decision to be considered not to have been made autonomously? This issue is often dealt with in legal cases. For the present it is enough to know that autonomy is compromised to the degree that coercion or undue influence impinge on the decision maker. If society seeks to promote autonomy, it must minimize these interferences. This was Mill's primary concern about autonomy.

The second source of constraints on autonomy is somewhat more difficult to deal with but no less important. Constraints arise within the individual, and philosophers have traditionally called them limitations on freedom of the will. This may seem an archaic term, but it refers to a real and important issue in autonomy in medical care. Persons who feel they are too stupid or too weak to make choices or who cannot find the emotional strength to do so are not capable of acting autonomously. As a result, they may become overly susceptible to influences that would otherwise not be considered undue. Because of the prestige of the medical profession and the status and deference accorded the professionals and experts in our society, it has been claimed, medical patients do not feel capable of making decisions for themselves (6, pp. 368–382). This position seems to hold that the entire doctrine of informed consent operates on a false premise and that therefore it cannot produce truly autonomous choices by patients. This black-and-white notion of autonomy represents an extreme stand. All actions are more or less free of constraints, more or less autonomous. Greater autonomy is a goal; complete autonomy is an unreachable (perhaps even undesirable) ideal (7,8).

It is also important, however, to understand what autonomy is *not* and thus what we are not obliged to respect if expressed by others. Autonomy does not mean doing whatever one might want to do. For Kant, autonomy consisted of persons' abilities to make their own rules and carry them out in behavior. These rules of behavior, to be ethical, had to be "universalizable"—that is, capable of being implemented by anyone in the same circumstances and yielding of results that are internally consistent.

Although many have felt that Kant's version of principled behavior is too restrictive, even Mill (the ultimate libertarian) restricted freedom of choice of behaviors to adults of sound mind and insisted that behavior not interfere with the rights of others. Autonomy does not come without obligations. For our purposes, this idea means that patients' rights to make medical decisions can in some circumstances be abrogated and should not be thought of as allowing patients to have whatever medical care they wish.

The Societal Grounding of Autonomy

Kant's ethical principles are couched in absolute terms. They are described as universally true or false. In our somewhat more cynical age it sometimes seems old-fashioned to speak of an absolute obligation not to treat another as a means to an end. However, precisely such principles are basic values of American society and form the moral foundations of a variety of institutions.

Sociologists often speak of *societal values*, or clusters of beliefs about what is desirable. At a general level these seem to be fairly stable over time within a society. Most sociologists identify a cluster of beliefs about the importance of the autonomy of the individual as the dominant set of values in American society. At the turn of the century, the French sociologist Emile Durkheim argued that the values of individualism were so dominant in Western culture as a whole that they functioned in much the same way as a religion—for example, to justify such basic institutional patterns as the doctor-patient relationship (9, p. 172). In other words, the promotion of individualism in general and the development of each individual in particular has become the almost sacred task of the society as a whole and of its members. Since Durkheim the roots of this particular value structure in our Judaic and Greek heritage have been explored, and Max Weber has written about the role of Protestant theology in the sanctification of the individual conscience (10, p. 8; 11). For both Weber and Durkheim, in somewhat different ways, the sanctification of the individual was the key to the development of a modern, highly differentiated social structure.

The sanctity of individual choice is used in our society to justify many practices, including the participation of patients in medical decision making, the core idea of informed consent. These are deontological justifications in the sense that the promotion of individual autonomy of patients is seen as a justifiable end in itself rather than promoting some other good end.

2.3 Deontological and Consequentialist Justifications of Informed Consent

The justification of informed consent as a central duty of healthcare professionals and as a right of patients follows from the deontological and consequentialist justifications of the principle of autonomy. Applied to the doctor-patient relationship, Kant's principle might require two behaviors by physicians. First, and most obviously, a physician must not engage in coercion in an attempt to compel patients to undergo particular medical procedures. Such coercion would undermine patients' abilities to pursue rational courses of action that are consistent with their ethical systems. The law has recognized the legitimacy of this principle for hundreds of years, deeming actions taken over patients' objections or without their free consent to constitute legally actionable intrusions on their bodily integrity. Few would quarrel with this conclusion, but defining unacceptable coercion in practice is, as has been noted, more difficult than this formulation suggests.

The second requirement derived from Kant's principle is a good deal more controversial. Rational decisionmaking can only be built on a foundation of accurate facts concerning a situation. If the physician, who is aware of the medical situation, fails to share such facts with the patient, who presumably is not, the latter will be unable to make a reasoned choice and therefore unable to act autonomously. Thus, the deontologic principle of autonomy requires that physicians provide to patients whatever information is necessary for their decision making, a key ethical grounding of the idea of informed consent. (How the law has elaborated on this requirement is described in Chapter 3, and an approach that integrates it into the doctor-patient relationship is detailed in Chapter 8.)

The consequentialist ethicist seeking to establish a basis for informed consent has, in some ways, a more difficult task than the deontologist, for consequentialism requires an assessment of likely outcomes, which are not always easy to identify. Consequentialists have not avoided the task, and their justifications of informed consent have the virtue of being more specific than many deontological ones. A general list of the benefits that might ensue from the idea of informed consent was compiled by Katz and Capron, who included among the functions of informed consent the following (12, pp. 82–90):

1. Promotion of individual autonomy
2. Protection of patients and subjects
3. Avoidance of fraud and duress
4. Encouragement of self-scrutiny by medical professionals
5. Promotion of rational decisions
6. Involvement of the public

Another analysis of the potential benefits of informed consent focused on the relationship between patients and their caregivers. In what has become one of the classic essays on the problems of the medical profession in America, Eliot Friedson suggested that what he views as the current dominance of the medical profession over the rest of the citizenry is essentially incompatible with a democratic society:

> It is often said these days that the world we live in has become so complex that it cannot survive unless it more and more comes to be ordered by the special technical knowledge of the expert or the professional. A recent paper celebrating the increasing importance of specialized knowledge in determining social policy refers to the decline of faith and politics in human affairs. Faith which all men may possess and politics in which all citizens participate fade away before knowledge

which only experts possess. . . . The relation of the expert to modern society seems in fact to be one of the central problems of our time, for at its heart lie the issues of democracy and freedom and the degree to which ordinary men can shape the character of their own lives (6, pp. 335–336).

For Friedson and many others, the practical consequences of true informed consent are the continuation of the democratic ideal and freedom from despotism of a new sort, the despotism of the expert (13, pp. 335–382).

At another extreme, a large group of social and behavioral scientists of medicine see informed consent as a tool to implement the same goals that medicine seeks to achieve. This group views the lack of patient participation in medical decisions not as a function of the medical profession's efforts to maintain its power, but as a reflection of the profession's ignorance of how vital patients' contribution can be to the shared goal of improving patients' health. In support of this position, research has shown that large numbers of patients do not comply with medical advice, particularly on preventive regimens that arguably are the key to improving the health of the general population. Stone has suggested that lack of patient participation in treatment decisions is a principle part of this problem (14). There is considerable empirical evidence for the view that the failure to explain treatment to patients is a major cause of patients' failure to comply (15).

Some see a more direct association between an individual's health and the nature of the doctor-patient relationship. For example, full disclosure to cancer patients may lead to less anxiety and depression, and there is ample evidence that such reactions are negatively correlated with positive health outcomes (16). Others combine a concern for compliance with an objection to non-democratic structures, suggesting that patients' noncompliance is actually a form of passive resistance to the practitioner's control of the relationship (17).

2.4 The Value of Autonomy versus the Value of Health

If autonomy were the only value to be taken into account in medical decision making, the idea of informed consent would be a good deal less controversial than it is. Most frequently seen as being in conflict with the value of autonomy is the value of health. This value, too, has both deontologic and consequentialist support, and there is no gainsaying its importance as an instinctual value even in primitive societies. From the religious deontologic point of view, the preservation of health can be seen as a means of honoring the Creator, whose handiwork reached a pinnacle in forming the human body. Religions as diverse as ancient Greek polytheism, Judaism, and Catholicism espouse this rationale for the promotion of health. In the secular context, preserving health can be seen as evidencing respect for humanity, particularly as rational beings. Consequentialists have an even easier time arguing the importance of health; not only is health itself a source of personal satisfaction, but it is a necessary prerequisite for the fulfillment of most other desires as well. Since healthy persons benefit their society—for example, in adding to the labor pool available for productive activity—the state may have an interest in promoting health even beyond the interest of any individual citizen.

It is noteworthy that when the societal interest in protecting health has come into conflict with the value of autonomy, the latter has often been forced to yield. Government exercises power to promote health, both to protect the interests of others under the police power, and to protect the individual under the *parens patriae* power (see below). These may be considered offshoots of the principles of nonmaleficence and beneficence, respectively.

In the realm of promoting health, a time-honored example of exercising the police power is compulsory quarantine laws that protect against the spread of contagious disease. Only the development of effective medical treatment for many contagious diseases has led to the repeal or desuetude of such laws, although their revitalization may be occurring in response to the problems of AIDS. A contemporary example of the exercise of the police power in the medical sphere is compulsory vaccination against contagious disease, a power that has been upheld by the United States Supreme Court (18). Perhaps an even more compelling example of the depth of society's commitment to the promotion of health at potential expense to individual liberty is the existence in every American jurisdiction of statutes for the involuntary civil commitment of those mentally disabled who are dangerous to others.

The fluoridation of public water supplies, the requirement that motorcyclists wear helmets, and statutes governing the involuntary civil commitment of the mentally disabled who are dangerous to themselves are three disparate examples of the exercise of the *parens patriae* power, in which the state acts for the benefit of the individual. More closely related to the concerns of this book is the ordering of involuntary rendition of medical treatment, especially blood transfusions. (See Chapters 4 and 5 for a further discussion of these cases.)

This position is diametrically opposed to autonomy, for in effect the state is saying, We know better than you what is best for you. This stance is not malevolent; quite the contrary, it is highly beneficent. It says to the person about to jump off a bridge that there is hope, that we do care, and that life might be better if it were given another chance; it says to the psychotic patient who refuses to take an antipsychotic medication that the medication will make the tormenting hallucinations go away; and it says to the person with a ruptured appendix who faces certain death unless operated upon, and refuses to undergo surgery because of fear of the minute risk of death from anesthesia, that fear has dictated the wrong decision.

Some critics of the idea of informed consent believe that the value of autonomy should be subordinated to the value of health in medical decision making in general. These commentators believe that encouraging patients to participate in decision making will promote rejection of needed treatment and cause patients needless psychological harm. (See Chapter 7.) It is argued that patients are unlikely to understand the information disclosed, and even if it is understood, unlikely to act on it.

In the development of the legal doctrine of informed consent, the law has been faced with the need to reconcile the competing values of autonomy and health. The result has been a divergence of the ideal model of informed consent—as the pure embodiment of the value of autonomy—from the legal requirements and rules for recovery created by courts. The reader will follow the thread of tension between autonomy and health through the rest of this book.

The courts have assumed a compromise position. They have accepted the arguments that autonomy can be antithetical to health to some extent, recognizing that there may be times when individual choice should be restricted. However, limitations on individual autonomy in medical decision making have come to be seen as the exception not the rule. The courts have sought to accommodate both values, realizing that the two can be at least partially complementary and need not detract from each other.

This compromise rests on the presumption that the primary decisional authority about medical treatment belongs to the patient, while the interest in promoting health is given its due in two different ways. First, certain of the rules for recovery (e.g., those defining the standards of disclosure and causation, discussed more fully in Chapter 6) limit the ability of patients to obtain redress for harms allegedly suffered as a result of inadequate disclosure of information. These rules in effect grant somewhat more discretion to physicians in shaping their disclosures, presumably with the goal of enhancing their influence over patients' decisions. Second, several exceptions to the general rule requiring disclosure and consent shift decisional authority away from patients under specified circumstances. These are generally cases when it is presumed that patients' exercise of this authority would cause more harm than good: in emergencies, when patients are incompetent, when they do not desire to be informed or to make decisions, or when the disclosure itself might harm them. (See Chapters 4 and 5.)

Some critics argue that informed consent law tilts too heavily to the side of individual autonomy, and others contend that attempts to promote health-related values have made autonomy meaningless. (See Chapter 7.) Our view is a middle-of-the-road position. We see the unified doctrine of informed consent—that is, the general rule and the exceptions taken together—as striking a balance in which the promotion of health is not inherently at odds with the allocation of primary decisional authority to the patient. Put somewhat differently, we believe that a reasonable approach to informed consent can be consistent both with good medical practice and with the ethical and legal theories.

References

1. Kant I: Metaphysical foundations of morals (C. S. Freidrich: trans.), in Beardsley M (ed.), *The European Philosophers*. New York, Modern Library, 1960.

2. Bentham J: An introduction to the principles of morals and legislation, in *The Utilitarians*. New York, Dolphin, 1961.

3. Mill JS: *On Liberty*. Chicago, H. Regnery, 1955.

4. Brandt RB: The real and alleged problems of utilitarianism, *Hastings Center Report*, 13(2):37–44, 1983.

5. National Commission for the Protection of Human Subjects of Biomedical and Behavioral Research: *The Belmont Report: Ethical Guidelines for the Protection of Human Subjects of Research*. DHEW Publication No. (OS) 78–0012. Washington, D.C., U.S. Government Printing Office, 1978.

6. Friedson E: *The Profession of Medicine*. New York, Dodd, Mead, 1970.

7. Brody H: Autonomy revisited: progress in medical ethics: discussion paper. *J Royal Soc Med* 78:380–387, 1985.

8. Callahan D: Autonomy: a moral good, not a moral obsession. *Hastings Center Report* 14(5):40–42, 1984.

9. Durkheim E: *The Division of Labor in Society*. Glencoe, Ill., The Free Press, 1933.

10. Parsons T: *Societies: Evolutionary and Comparative Perspectives*. Englewood Cliffs, N.J., Prentice-Hall, 1966.

11. Weber M: *The Protestant Ethic and the Spirit of Capitalism*. New York, Scribner's, 1958, passim.

12. Katz J, Capron AM: *Catastrophic Diseases: Who Decides What?* New York, Russell Sage Foundation, 1975.

13. Illich I: *Medical Nemesis: The Expropriation of Health*. New York, Pantheon Books, 1982.

14. Stone GC: Patient compliance and the role of the expert. *Journal of Social Issues* 35:34–59, 1979.

15. Francis V, Korsch BM, Morris MJ: Gaps in doctor-patient communications: patients' response to medical advice. *N Engl J Med* 280:535–540, 1969.

16. Gerle B, Lundin G, Sandblom P: The patient with inoperable cancer from the psychiatric and social standpoint. *Cancer* 13:1206–1217, 1960.

17. Waitzkin H, Stoeckle J: The communication of information about illness. *Adv Psychosom Med* 8:180–215, 1972.

18. Jacobson v. Massachusetts, 197 U.S. 11 (1905).

II

THE LEGAL THEORY OF
INFORMED CONSENT

3

The Legal Requirements
for Disclosure and Consent:
History and Current Status

The translation of ethical principles into concrete requirements for physicians' behavior has been largely a function of the courts (usually state, occasionally federal) as they consider patients' allegations that their physicians improperly obtained their consent to treatment. State legislatures to a lesser extent have been involved in making law in this area. The combined efforts of courts and legislatures have resulted in the creation of two legal requirements: the historic requirement that physicians obtain patients' consent before proceeding with treatment, and the more recent requirement that physicians disclose such information to patients as will enable them to participate intelligently in making decisions about treatment. (Chapters 4 and 5 describe the exceptional circumstances in which some or all of the basic legal requirements do not apply.)

3.1 The Historical Context

Despite some uncertainty about the origins of legal actions for lack of consent to medical treatment, in theory nonconsensual medical treatment has always been remediable at common law. Law's concern for the bodily integrity of the individual—that is, its embodiment of the ethical principle of autonomy—can be traced to the writ of trespass for assault and battery and to the criminal law proscription of homicide, battery, and mayhem (1, p. 312). A similar, though less intense, concern for psychic integrity has existed for almost as long and has received increasing support in this century in the cases recognizing causes of action in tort law for intentional infliction of emotional distress (2, pp. 8–11; 3, §12; 4, §46). Similarly, the development of the constitutional and tort law of privacy reflects the continued vitality of society's concern for the individual's right to be let alone, both by agents of the state (3, §54) and by private parties (5, pp. 886–990).

The historic legal rule is that physicians must obtain their patients' consent before they are legally entitled to commence treatment. The first reported case to have applied this rule was the late eighteenth-century English case of *Slater* v. *Baker & Stapleton*, which held two medical practitioners liable for disuniting, without the patient's consent, a partially healed fracture (6). What is most interesting about this case is that it seemed to predicate the legal requirement for consent not merely upon the, even then, time-honored rule that the nonconsensual and unprivileged touching of another person's body is a battery, but upon the fact that it was the custom of surgeons not to operate on patients without their consent:

> [I]t appears from the evidence of the surgeons that it was improper to disunite the callous without consent; this is the usage and law of surgeons: then it was ignorance and unskillfulness in that very particular, to do contrary to the rule of the profession, what no surgeon ought to have done (6).

Besides constituting a recognition of the ethical and legal requirements of consent, this professional custom was probably also based on the need for the patient's cooperation if surgery were to be performed without the use of an anesthetic, as was then necessary. Despite this statement of the court, there is a good deal of evidence to suggest that physicians historically saw the requirements for consent as minimal, requiring that little or no information be disclosed before permission to proceed was obtained. Even some distortion of the facts was tolerated in the name of encouraging patients' compliance and cooperation.

The *Slater* court made some interesting observations on the role of communication in the doctor-patient relationship that might be taken as rudimentary precursors of the consequentialist justifications of informed consent. Not only was it customary for the surgeon to obtain the patient's consent, the court observed, but "indeed it is reasonable that a patient should be told what is about to be done to him that he may take courage and put himself in such a situation as to enable him to undergo the operation"(6).

By the early 1900s, cases raising questions about the legal authority of physicians to render treatment began to occur with some frequency in the United States. The paucity of such cases prior to the beginning of this century says as much about the previously restricted societal role of the medical profession as it says about the equally restricted role of litigation as a means of resolving disputes. However, even when such cases began to arise, courts were willing to find that patients had not provided valid consent to treatment only in the clearest circumstances. A simple interchange between patient and physician long passed for valid consent. In substance, the physician said to the patient, "You need thus-and-so to get better," and the patient responded with some phrase or action indicating the intention to go along with the doctor's recommendations or not. The response may have been very broad: O.K. Doc, whatever you say; slightly less inclusive: Go ahead and do thus-and-so; somewhat more limiting: Go ahead and do *thus*, but I don't want you to do any *so* (7–10); or even totally restrictive: If that's what I need, then I'd rather be sick, and don't do anything at all (7–13).

Each of these responses (even the express prohibition!) has been considered authorization to treat by physicians at various times. The courts have generally agreed that the patient has, by speaking some such phrase (except the express prohibition), authorized the physician to proceed and thereby provided the physician with a defense to an action for battery.

It was not until the beginning of the twentieth century that litigation over the requirement of consent to medical treatment began in earnest. Slowly the realization grew that an authorization for treatment consistent with the principle of autonomy might be

more complicated than it originally seemed (14, p. 789). For example, the doctor might not have merely said, "You need thus-
and-so to get better," but (trying to put an anxious patient at ease)
might have added, "Oh, it's not a serious operation at all." The
patient might then have agreed to undergo the procedure, much
assured that it was a simple operation, and been distraught at the
conclusion of the operation when undesirable results were discovered (15–18).

A more complicated set of rules began to develop beyond the
original simple proposition that a physician might not treat a patient without the patient's authorization. Not only was the physician required to obtain the patient's consent to treatment, but if
the physician affirmatively misrepresented the nature of the procedure and the probable consequences, the misrepresentation
might be held to invalidate the patient's consent, leaving the physician open to a claim for unauthorized treatment (13,15,17–20).
The courts uniformly held that fraudulent, deceptive, or misleading
disclosure vitiated the consent that the patient subsequently gave
(15–18).

This early rule—that ordinarily no information need be provided, but if the physician did provide information, it must be
truthful—contained the seeds of the requirement of an affirmative
duty of disclosure. While several cases before the middle of the
twentieth century intimated that this duty existed, they were
greatly scattered both temporally and geographically and even in
retrospect do not constitute any coherent pattern (15,22,23).

The Transition From Simple to Informed Consent

A group of cases in the 1950s marks a clear transition from the
older simple consent rule to the first contemporary informed consent cases. In 1955, the Supreme Court of North Carolina stated
that the failure to explain the risks involved in surgery "may be
considered a mistake on the part of the surgeon" (16). In *Salgo*
v. *Leland Stanford Jr. University Board of Trustees* two years later,
a California court—relying in part on the North Carolina precedent—specifically held that physicians had an affirmative duty of
disclosure to enable patients to provide an "informed" consent
(21). The court, however, failed to offer a detailed and explicit

statement of what kinds of information the affirmative duty of disclosure entailed. A jury verdict for the plaintiff was actually reversed on appeal, on the ground that the trial court's instruction on the duty to inform went further than required.

The following year, the Supreme Court of Minnesota reinforced the affirmative duty of disclosure. It held a physician liable for failing to inform a patient before surgery of alternative forms of treatment that would not have entailed the undesirable consequence of the procedure actually performed (24).

While some courts at this time were imposing an affirmative duty of disclosure upon physicians, others were reiterating the older view that physicians had no such duty (25,26). One court even imposed liability upon a physician for mental anguish caused by information that he disclosed to the patient about her condition and its proper treatment (27).

The Doctrine Defined

The most significant of the cases in the mid–1950s is probably *Salgo* (21), primarily because it coined the term informed consent. A patient who had undergone transthoracic aortography—a now outmoded technique of puncturing the aorta through the back, in order to inject radio-opaque dye—suffered paralysis of the legs, a rare but not unheard-of complication. The jury should be instructed, said the court, that "the physician has . . . discretion [to withhold alarming information from the patient] consistent, of course, with the full disclosure of facts necessary to an informed consent" (21).

Despite the use of this new term, *Salgo* did not advance the developing law a great deal. In fact, as Katz has cogently observed, the case contributed substantially to the confusion that already existed and continues to exist about the requirements of the informed consent doctrine in its attempt to reconcile two inherently contradictory terms: "Only in dreams or fairy tales," he wrote, "can 'discretion' to withhold crucial information so easily and magically be reconciled with 'full disclosure' " (28). Nevertheless, *Salgo* did provide a certain stability to the notion of a duty to disclose by coining the term informed consent, a handy—if facile— means of describing the evolving legal requirement.

It took another three years for the courts to begin systematically to sketch in the contours of the doctrine. Two cases (decided in different jurisdictions within two days of each other) in 1960 clearly indicated that there was to be no turning back from the imposition of an affirmative duty of disclosure. Judicial movement beyond the simple consent requirement had been in the air during the 1950s, but the decisions in *Natanson* v. *Kline* and *Mitchell* v. *Robinson* made it clear that the simple ways of the past would no longer suffice (29,30).

In *Natanson*, a woman had suffered substantial burns to the thorax from radiation therapy performed after a mastectomy. In *Mitchell*, the plaintiff received insulin shock and electroshock therapy for the treatment of schizophrenia, causing the fracture of several vertebrae. In both cases the patients' consents to treatment had been obtained. However, they asserted that the physicians had had an affirmative duty to them to disclose information about the risks of the treatment, that this duty had not been fulfilled, and that the breach constituted negligence. Both courts agreed. The *Mitchell* court phrased the duty as requiring the physician "to inform [the patient] generally of the possible serious collateral hazards" (30). The *Natanson* court went further, describing the doctor's duty as requiring

> a reasonable disclosure... of the nature and probable consequences of the suggested or recommended... treatment, and... a reasonable disclosure of the dangers within his knowledge which were incident to, or possible in, the treatment he proposed to administer (29).

Mitchell and *Natanson* both held that the central information that needed to be disclosed was the possible bad results of a particular procedure. This concept, which has been expressed in several ways—side-effects, collateral hazards, dangers, perils—is generally referred to as the *risks* of the procedure. It is self-evident that if persons are to make informed, autonomous choices, they must be told not only that the procedures are intended to diagnose or treat the condition from which they suffer, but also that the procedures may fail to do so, or that they may be worse off after the procedures. Disclosure of risks does not guarantee that patients will utilize the information or that their decisions will be reasonable. Yet without this information most patients are unable to make the kind of informed decisions that are central to the ethical notion of autonomous choice.

While *Mitchell* mandated only the disclosure of risk information, *Natanson,* as noted, went further, requiring disclosure of the nature of the ailment, the nature of the proposed treatment, the probability of success, and possible alternative treatments. These requirements, with slight modifications of terminology, are now the bedrock elements of the information that the informed consent cases and statutes require physicians to provide to patients.

Merely specifying the type of information that must be disclosed to patients did not obviate the need for further clarification. Physicians were well aware that all medications and most procedures, even simple ones, carry risks that range from minor to life-threatening and vary in frequency from omnipresent to rare. Which of these many risks were physicians now obligated to disclose? Similarly, how much information about the nature of the procedure and how many alternatives were physicians required to discuss? The jurisprudence of informed consent in the years since *Natanson* and *Mitchell* has addressed these issues in considerable detail.

3.2 Standards of Disclosure

Professional Standards

In the formative years of the legal doctrine of informed consent— the 1950s and 1960s—the courts held that the degree of disclosure made to patients was primarily a question of medical judgment. Consequently, "[t]he duty of the physician to disclose . . . is limited to those disclosures which a reasonable medical practitioner would make under the same or similar circumstances" (29). This rule of recovery closely parallels the rules of recovery in medical negligence (or malpractice) cases generally: Physicians are held to the standard of what is customary and usual in the profession, not only in the exercise of skill, but also in the disclosure of information to patients (31;32,¶8.04). The courts of numerous jurisdictions explicitly adopted this rule, and few seriously questioned it for more than a decade (33).

The advantages of a professional (or customary) standard, as this approach came to be called, include the legal system's familiarity with it, and the fact that the freedom of the medical profession (as a whole—not necessarily the freedom of the individual physician) to shape the contours of appropriate disclosure is maintained. If one believes that doctors generally—perhaps as a result of dealing with many patients over the years—know how much a patient should be told about a medical procedure, depending both on what factors are objectively important and what issues seem to be of greatest concern to the patient, the professional standard is both acceptable and desirable. In addition, it places no extra burden on physicians to conform to an externally imposed standard, since they presumably already know about and observe professional norms.

However, three problems with the use of a professional standard quickly became apparent. First, as Judge Robinson remarked in the landmark case of *Canterbury* v. *Spence*, it is not at all certain for many medical procedures that there is "any discernible custom reflecting a professional concensus [sic] on communication of option and risk information to patients" about recommended treatment (31). In other words, in cases where there is no professional custom of disclosing, the legal right to obtain information is undermined by professional practice.

Second, even where professional standards exist they may be set too low to satisfy the needs of patients who wish to participate in medical decision making in accord with the idea of informed consent. For example, the custom of physicians may be to inform patients of only the minor risks of a particular procedure, so as not to frighten off patients from receiving treatment. Although the motivation may be to help patients in accord with what physicians view as their patients' best interests, this degree of restriction on disclosure utterly vitiates the purpose of informed consent. In addition, even a standard of fairly complete disclosure of information *physicians* believe to be important does not offer recourse to a patient who believes injury occurred because information most *patients* would want to know was not revealed.

Third, in cases where professional standards are used, the plaintiff must obtain an expert witness, in this instance a physician familiar with the relevant subject matter, to establish the standard of care (34). This procedure is the norm in most medical malpractice cases, the only exception being when the issue at question is within the reasonable knowledge of laypersons. (For example, if a surgeon leaves a sponge or an instrument in the abdominal cavity, a court will permit the jury to find that this conduct does not constitute reasonable care even without an expert witness.) Thus in informed consent cases the requirement was imposed on the plaintiff of presenting an expert to establish what reasonable practitioners would disclose.

For a variety of reasons, this proved to be as onerous a requirement as it had long been in other kinds of malpractice cases (33). A plaintiff's primary difficulty in obtaining an expert witness was the unwillingness of physicians to testify against other physicians (35). This obstacle is often reduced if the plaintiff is permitted to seek out a physician who practices in another city, county, or state. However, in the 1960s and early 1970s, many courts held firm to an old rule known as the locality rule: to establish the standard of care in a malpractice case, the plaintiff had to use an expert witness familiar with the standard of practice in the defendant-doctor's own locality. In fact, the standard of care to which a physician was held was that of a reasonably prudent physician practicing in the defendant's locality. The rationale was that it was manifestly unfair to hold physicians to standards of practice that their geographic isolation and limited resources might not permit them to attain.

Because of improved transportation and communication and a growing belief within the profession that standards need not be disparate, the rationale for the locality rule has eroded and it has gone into decline (36). Nevertheless, a number of courts still adhere to it, some informed consent legislation also employs it (37), and it occasionally continues to be applied in informed consent cases (34).

While the vitality of the locality rule has diminished, it is still not always easy for plaintiffs to obtain the testimony of experts. At the very least, the need for such testimony continues to be a hurdle patients must surmount to obtain compensation in professional-standard jurisdictions.

Patient-Oriented Standards

With these considerations in mind, within a matter of months in 1971 and 1972 a number of courts substantially challenged the slightly more than 10-year-old rule regarding the professional standard of disclosure (31,38–40). Because there may be no custom in the medical profession to disclose information to patients, because disclosure of information "does not bring [the physician's special] medical knowledge and skills peculiarly into play" (31), and because of the difficulty in obtaining expert witnesses, these courts rejected the professional standard of disclosure. In its place they required that physicians disclose as much information as a *patient* would want to know. (Which patient to use as the benchmark arose immediately as an important issue.) This new formulation of the standard of care was variously referred to as a lay, legal, or patient-oriented standard—lay, because the adequacy of disclosure was applied by laypersons (jurors) unaided by expert witnesses; legal, because it was imposed by courts rather than by medical custom; and patient-oriented because its aim was that patients be provided with information that would enable them to make intelligent choices.

The adoption of patient-oriented standards was motivated in part by the lack of professional standards and by plaintiffs' difficulties obtaining expert witnesses. However, the fundamental motivation was the assumption that the underlying rationale of the informed consent doctrine is to permit patients to exercise choice concerning the risks to which they are willing to subject themselves. Thus, the *Canterbury* court, in the leading opinion among these cases, concluded that "[r]espect for the patient's right of self-determination on particular therapy demands a standard set by law for physicians rather than one which physicians may or may not impose upon themselves" (31). To permit physicians to determine what information is to be disclosed by reference either to their own personal standards or to standards of the medical profession is to undercut the right of patients to have information available that they might find relevant to the decisions they must make.

This last point is particularly important because it reflects a recognition that the informed consent requirement goes beyond the older, simple consent requirement in the interests that it protects. The purpose of the simple consent requirement—protecting patients from unwanted interferences with their bodily integrity—was important, but limited in comparison with the purpose of informed consent, which is additionally to permit patients to make choices about their health care.

A fair statement of the rule that emerged is that the physician is required to disclose all information about a proposed treatment that a reasonable person in the patient's circumstances would find material to a decision either to undergo or forego treatment (31). The scope of the duty to disclose is to be determined by what is called the patient's right to decide, not by the custom or practice of either the particular physician or the larger medical profession.

The patient-oriented standard of disclosure was rapidly adopted by the courts. Between 1970, when it was formulated by Waltz and Scheuneman (41), and 1978 about half the courts considering the issue moved in this direction. Since then, however, there has been a gradual reverse trend, and at this time a small majority of states still adhere to the professional standard of disclosure (42).

The patient-oriented standard imposes upon physicians more substantial obligations than does the professional standard. Assuming that it actually is the custom of the profession to make disclosure to patients (this assumption is questionable (43), and has not been and probably now cannot be, investigated in a scientific fashion) physicians have reasonably ready ways of knowing what the standard is and of complying with it. Medical education and supervised clinical training, formal continuing education, and informal discourse among colleagues all help to inform physicians as to what it is customary to tell patients about treatment. For the same reasons that the content of the standard is easily accessible to physicians, it is relatively simple to establish in a trial, assuming that other physicians are willing to serve as expert witnesses.

By comparison, the content of the patient-oriented standard is especially difficult for physicians to ascertain. The professional standard is factual and therefore empirically determinable; the patient-oriented standard is hypothetical. It requires physicians to disclose the information that a reasonably prudent person would find material to making a decision. The reasonably prudent person of tort law is a hypothetical construct used by the fact finders—usually jurors, in informed consent cases—to develop and apply what they perceive to be community standards of reasonable conduct. After a particular kind of problem is litigated, more concrete standards may begin to evolve—more rapidly, the more frequently it is litigated. But within very broad limits the jury is free to write on a clean slate. Previous jury verdicts are not binding precedent. In every case, the jury is required to determine what is reasonable disclosure, taking into account all the facts and circumstances of the particular case.

The very difficulty in knowing and applying the patient-oriented standard turns out to be its virtue (though possibly not from physicians' perspective). To determine what a reasonable patient would find material to making a decision, physicians are compelled to engage in a discussion with each patient. In so doing, they act to implement one of the fundamental goals of the idea of informed consent: to involve patients in decision making about their own care.

This, of course, is an idealized version of how informed consent operates under the patient-oriented standard. Empirical evidence in support of this model is lacking; in fact, there is some evidence to the contrary (43). The fact that so few patients sue physicians in general, even fewer sue claiming lack of informed consent, and yet fewer prevail on that theory, along with the absence of any other effective enforcement mechanisms, means that in practice the patient-oriented standard may differ little in its impact on disclosure practices from the professional standard. It is even possible that physicians can ignore the informed consent requirement, regardless of the standard, with relative impunity from legal consequences. What little evidence there is suggests that this may be the case (44,45).

It has been argued that even the patient-oriented standard as formulated in *Canterbury* is not entirely adequate to making the legal requirements true to the idea of informed consent. To the extent that informed consent is intended to permit patients to make medical decisions based on their own personal beliefs, values, and goals, even the patient-oriented standard, as applied by the overwhelming proportion of courts, undermines this objective. This standard requires physicians to tell patients what a reasonable person would find material to making a decision—hence its designation as an objective standard. It therefore compels a particular patient whose values differ from the norm to be satisfied with the quantum of information dictated by that norm. A patient who works as a watch repairer, for example, may be very interested to know that a medication occasionally causes a fine tremor, whereas to most patients—hence to the hypothetical reasonable patient—such information would be of little importance. If a particular patient needs information that most patients would not find useful or necessary, there may be no legal entitlement to that information unless the patient specifically asks for it or the physician knows or should have reason to know of the patient's particularized need.

A very small number of courts and legislatures have recognized this deficiency in the objective patient-oriented standard and applied as a remedy a *subjective* patient-oriented standard (42,46). Under this standard, a physician is obligated to disclose the information that the *particular* patient would find material to making a decision about treatment. Thus, the standard is subjective and personal to each patient. In order to determine what the patient needs to know to make a decision, the physician is compelled even more than under the objective patient-oriented standard to engage in a conversation with the patient about treatment.

Mixed Standards

The distinction between professional and patient-oriented standards offers a useful dialectic for conceptual purposes, but in practice the boundary between these two categories is often blurred. The decision in *Natanson* v. *Kline*, for example, is frequently cited as the paradigmatic example of the adoption of a professional standard for disclosure (29). The term professional standard as applied to the case, however, is something of a misnomer. The *Natanson* court attempted to keep the newly defined duty to obtain informed consent within the bounds of traditional negligence law by referring to the behavior of a "reasonable medical practitioner," but the opinion went further than this phrase suggests. Apparently recognizing the unlikeliness of the medical profession disclosing much information to patients at the time, the court itself defined the framework within which medical discretion might operate (47). The court not only described the areas the physician's disclosure was required to cover (the nature of the illness and proposed treatment, the probability of success and of "unfortunate results and unforeseen consequences," and the alternative treatments available), but also required that the disclosure be "sufficient to insure an informed consent," and that it be made "in language as

simple as necessary." These terms represented a potentially significant limitation on the medical profession's capacity to set its
own standards. If the usual medical practice were to explain op-
erations to patients in highly technical terms, or to limit disclosure
severely, this would presumably not provide an adequate defense
to a charge of negligence under *Natanson*.

The approach of the *Natanson* court might better be called a
"modified professional standard" (48). It is as if the court were
saying, "So long as you physicians operate within the parameters
of behavior that we consider reasonable in relation to disclosure,
we will allow you to set the precise standards yourselves. If you
deviate from the broad outlines that we have in mind, we may be
compelled to intervene and establish standards of our own." As
in *Natanson*, courts do from time to time assume the power to
establish reasonable standards of professional or commercial practice when they believe that an entire profession or industry has
been derelict in monitoring its practices (49,50). Despite the failure
of the opinion in *Natanson* to own up to this approach, it is clear
that in significant part this is the course it took.

To be sure, certain courts and state legislatures have adopted
genuine professional standards of disclosure. In *Bly* v. *Rhoads*, for
example, the Virginia Supreme Court required plaintiffs to show
"that prevailing medical practice requires disclosure of certain information" and did not limit professional practices in any way (34).
Thus, the professional standard really embodies two different
standards, one a pure approach looking to professional self-reg-
ulation, and one a mixed model. The first leaves the issue of disclosure entirely in medical hands, while the second establishes the
boundaries within which medical opinion may be determinative.

Another type of mixed standard should be mentioned as well.
LeBlang has noted a tendency for some courts to combine the
professional and patient-oriented standards by requiring disclosure
to meet both standards (51). That is, if information were withheld
that either professional practices or the desires of a reasonable
patient would indicate should be disclosed, liability could be imposed. Although LeBlang calls this a "hybrid" standard, it seems
likely that in practice it would have the same effect as the more
demanding of its components, the patient-oriented standard; it
would be an odd court that would rule that the professional stan-

dard was not subsumed by the patient-oriented standard—that is, that anything physicians ordinarily disclose is not material to the decision of a reasonable person.

3.3 Elements of Disclosure: Further Guidance for Physicians

Standards of disclosure are intended to address the question, How much information must patients be given? If the answers to this question provided by courts and legislatures do not seem particularly helpful in assisting physicians to understand the extent of their obligations to reveal information to patients, this may be explained in part by the fact that these standards are derived from the requirements of the litigation process. They are devised not to aid physicians in performing their legal duty to inform patients, but to instruct juries in deciding in retrospect whether or not a particular defendant-physician had adequately informed the patient-plaintiff.

Judicial opinions and legislative enactments have addressed a related question: What information must patients be given? The answer frequently provided has been that for a patient to be adequately informed by legal standards, information must be given about the nature and purpose of the proposed treatment, its risks and benefits, and any available alternatives. These have come to be known as the *elements* of disclosure. Again, the goal of the courts in addressing this issue has largely been to assist juries rather than instruct physicians.

Nonetheless, these are not unrelated goals, and it is possible to glean from the enormous body of case law and statutes some basic guidelines for the proper scope of physicians' disclosures. Although differences among states cannot be ignored, certain generalizations can be extracted from the opinions and statutes that should be useful to all clinicians. Inevitably, there will be courts that disagree with these generalizations. The conclusions that follow, insofar as they represent an attempt to anticipate how courts will interpret the required elements and standards of disclosure in a given case, must be seen as suggested guidelines, not concrete rules.

Nature of the Procedure

Many courts and legislatures explicitly require that the nature of the procedure be explained to patients in order for a physician to obtain their informed consent. Of course, this requirement is no novelty, since the historic simple consent standard was based on disclosure of the nature of the treatment to be performed. Frequently the requirement is coupled with one to disclose the "character" of the treatment (52) or its "purpose" (53). Sometimes there is the qualification that the patient must have a "true understanding" of the nature of the procedure (54).

There are several different ways in which the nature of a medical procedure may be conceptualized. When a procedure is diagnostic rather than therapeutic, that fact ought to be explained, since the ordinary expectation of patients is likely to be that physicians' ministrations are meant to bring relief from suffering. Further, patients should be told whether a procedure is invasive—that is, whether it involves physical entry into their body (e.g., angiography) or not (e.g., chest x-ray). Other often relevant aspects include the duration of the treatment, the location where it will take place, the need for anesthesia, the sorts of instruments to be used, and an explanation of the bodily parts affected by the procedure. Many patients are concerned about exposure to radiation; the use of radiation and some rough way of quantifying its magnitude (e.g., "about as much as a chest x-ray") may be an important part of describing the procedure. The fact that a procedure is experimental or part of a research protocol is also essential to the nature of the procedure.

Risks

The element of information most heavily emphasized in the common law and statutory law of informed consent is risks. This emphasis is far out of proportion to that given other elements of disclosure. Katz has observed that the idea of informed consent envisioned by courts in their opinions has degenerated to little more than a duty to warn about risks (28,54). In actual medical practice, the requirement to obtain informed consent is often implemented in such a way as to focus on risk disclosure almost to the exclusion of other important information.

To determine which risks must be disclosed, a physician must refer to the prevailing standard of disclosure. The courts and legislatures often refer to and distinguish among material, substantial, probable, and significant risks (37), and these modifiers are not always easy to apply. Thus, in a certain state it may be acknowledged that risks must be disclosed, but the physician must engage in considerable thought relative to the prevailing standard of disclosure to determine whether disclosure of a particular risk must be made.

Although courts have not attempted any substantial analysis of the meaning of the term "risk," it can be inferred from the opinions on the subject that a physician needs to consider four separate aspects of risk in determining what information to disclose. These are (1) the nature of the risk, (2) the magnitude of the risk, (3) the probability that the risk might materialize, and (4) the imminence of risk materialization. If, for example, the risk of a particular procedure is that it may sever nerves that control movement of a limb, the nature of the risk is just that: the loss of motion in that appendage. The nature of a risk is important in determining whether or not a patient contemplating the procedure in question should be told about it, but it will not resolve the issue.

The magnitude, or seriousness, of the risk is a closely related factor. Analysis of the magnitude is often straightforward—loss of movement in a limb, blindness, or death are serious sequelae for any patient. Sometimes, on the other hand, one must consider the interaction between the nature of the risk and the situation of a particular patient. A minor loss of sensation in the hand may not be terribly serious for a retiree whose main occupation is watching television, but could be critical to a retiree who is an amateur sculptor.

The probability of a risk being manifested must also be taken into account. Even the fact that a risk is very serious (e.g., paraplegia, blindness, death) does not necessarily mean that it must be disclosed. If the probability is extremely low, nondisclosure may be justifiable. Similarly, if a risk is fairly likely to occur but relatively minor, nondisclosure may again be justifiable.

Finally, a patient may wish to consider the imminence of the risk—that is, when the risk might materialize, if it will materialize at all. A risk that is likely to occur immediately postoperatively, for example, may be considered more serious by some patients than a risk that materializes gradually or one that materializes after the passage of a substantial period of time.

Another related matter is what we call the problem of *lesser included* risks. A physician may believe that because patients have been informed about a particularly serious risk of a procedure, there is no need to inform them about less serious risks. The difficulty with this apparently logical view, particularly in a jurisdiction applying a patient-oriented standard, is that what is more or less serious is a subjective matter. A physician may believe that because a patient has been told the removal of a spinal tumor could lead to death, there is no need to discuss the possibility that it may also result in paraplegia. However, this particular patient may fear the latter far more than the former, and a jury may conclude that a reasonable person informed about the possibility of death would wish to know about the possibility of paraplegia as well (55–58).

In some states, statutes are very specific and require that only certain risks, such as those of "brain damage, quadriplegia, paraplegia, the loss or loss of function of any organ or limb, or disfiguring scars" be enumerated, even though they may have a very low probability (37). In these states the physician need not disclose other possible risks to obtain an informed consent. In effect, those enumerated are deemed material as a matter of law.

Texas adopted this checklist approach to the fullest extent. A panel of physicians and lawyers was statutorily established to develop a list of procedures and the risks which must be disclosed for each, and another list of procedures for which no disclosure need be made (59). The Hawaii statutory scheme relies upon an administrative agency to establish the scope of the required disclosure, defined as "reasonable medical standards, applicable to specific treatment and surgical procedures" (60).

Such systems may lend greater precision to the task of disclosure but they are contrary to the spirit of the informed consent doctrine. Their effect is to depersonalize the physician-patient relationship rather than to emphasize the necessity for increased communication in the name of enhancing patient autonomy. This is a serious problem. The practice of medicine has itself become increasingly technological and impersonal. If communication between physician and patient is to be based on the same model, patients may have even less knowledge about and control over the care they receive. Under this wooden approach, it might be possible to have a computer make the necessary disclosure to the patient, in much the same way that computers are now being programmed to make medical diagnoses. In fact, after a computer makes a diagnosis, it could also be programmed to make the appropriate disclosure for the recommended procedure (61).

Another technique courts and legislatures have used to define the boundaries of the scope of the required disclosure is to set forth certain risks that need *not* be disclosed. This category, called commonly known risks, is frequently mentioned. The rationale is that patients should be required to bring into the physician's office the common sense that the law expects them to exercise generally for their own well-being. Some courts have evaluated whether a certain risk is commonly known in terms of a subjective test. Thus, judge or jury must consider whether the risk in question was "in fact known to the patient usually because of a past experience with the procedure in question" (39). But in other jurisdictions that recognize commonly known risks as outside the scope of required disclosure, the formulation of the test has been an objective one, based on the knowledge of a reasonable patient.

In some jurisdictions, the statutes and cases also explicitly provide that so-called remote or minor risks need not be disclosed (37). The term remote seems to refer to those risks bearing a low probability, or in more conventional legal terminology, those risks that are not reasonably foreseeable. In contrast, the term minor seems to refer to the nature or magnitude of harm, rather than likelihood. Minor risks are those which, if they materialize, will not cause the patient substantial harm, pain, or discomfort.

We refer to these types of information that need not be disclosed—common, known, remote, or minor risks—as negative elements of disclosure. Alternatively, they may be viewed merely as concrete applications of the standard of disclosure, and even those jurisdictions that do not make specific provision for them are likely to recognize them in appropriate circumstances. That is, the negative elements need not be disclosed because under a lay standard of disclosure, as a matter of law, a reasonable patient would not find them material to medical decision making simply *because* they are remote or minor or known. And under a professional standard of disclosure, they need not be disclosed because it is not customary for physicians to tell patients about risks of which, for example, the patient is already aware (i.e., known risks). Thus, even in those jurisdictions that do not specifically recognize the negative elements, it can be said with a high degree of certainty that they need not be disclosed.

Alternatives or Options

Although less frequently recognized by courts and legislatures, a patient's knowledge of alternatives to recommended treatment is as important, possibly more important, to medical decision making than knowledge of risks. The notion of options is central to the idea of informed consent (62).

The term alternatives suggests that the physician has already determined what is best for the patient, and that any other procedures are secondary in value. In one sense, this is true. Physicians ought to suggest what they deem to be the medically preferable course. However, if decision making about care were simply a matter of what is preferable on medical grounds alone, there would be no need for the informed consent doctrine; simple consent would do just as well if not better. The physician would propose the medically preferable course of treatment, and the patient would decide to have it or not. The idea of informed consent is premised on the assumption that decision making about medical care should take account of patients' values, preferences, goals, and needs. Perfectly reasonable people may choose a course of medical care that is less than optimal as measured by medical criteria, and this choice is required by legal and ethical considerations to be respected.

When viewed in this light, the decision involves choosing among medically acceptable options, not simply accepting or rejecting the medically preferable option (31). For patients to make such choices, they must be informed about the nature and purpose of options, as well as their risks and benefits. They will then presumably be able to evaluate the comparative medical risks and benefits in light of their personal considerations. For these reasons it may make more sense to speak of options than alternatives, although the terms are often used interchangeably.

There are some medical procedures for which there are no reasonable alternatives. In most cases, however, options can be identified. Often the choice among options is merely a matter of medical taste and may be influenced by the specialty of a particular doctor. There may be no objective standard for determining that one procedure is preferable to another. In any case, there is always the alternative of no treatment. Despite the importance of the concept of alternatives in informed decision making, the requirement that they be disclosed is sometimes absent in case law and statutes (63).

Benefits

Occasionally a court or legislature has stated that in making proper disclosure a physician is obliged to enumerate the treatment's expected benefits. In most instances, the anticipated benefits are self-evident and probably the same as the purpose of the procedure—to relieve or remove the problem that occasioned the patient's seeking treatment. The patient is suffering from some illness or injury and anticipates that the proposed procedure will relieve that suffering. In such an instance, failure to disclose expressly the anticipated benefits is not so important.

There are, however, two situations in which benefit disclosure is crucial. First, when the procedure is diagnostic rather than therapeutic, the patient should be explicitly informed that it is not intended to relieve suffering directly, but only to provide information as to whether and how therapeutic procedures might be initiated. Second, in all instances in which the anticipated benefits are something less than full relief of the patient's suffering, the physician should inform the patient of that limitation. In this regard, the concept of benefits bears a close conceptual relationship to that of risks, the risk being the probability of a less than complete cure. Thus, the provision of information with a negative connotation, rather than the positive connotation we ordinarily associate with the term benefits, may also be required in order to fulfill the duty of disclosure.

Summary of the Requirements of Disclosure

The law of informed consent has developed almost exclusively from cases in which injured patients have claimed that a physician failed adequately to inform them before they consented to treatment. The primary aim of the judicial opinions in these cases has been to create a workable structure within which patients may obtain compensation for their injuries when there was lack of informed consent. The judicial opinions explain to judges and lawyers how such cases are to be litigated—what the plaintiff-patient must prove and how it must be proved in order to recover damages from the defendant-physician, and what affirmative defenses might be available to the physician if in fact adequate information was not conveyed to the patient. Only secondarily have the courts been concerned with instructing physicians on how informed consent is to be obtained.

Even those parts of judicial opinions that deal with the broader aspects of informed consent are not particularly helpful in instructing physicians. This lack of helpfulness arises in part from the sweeping generalities of the opinions. Even when courts do attend more specifically to explaining to doctors what constitutes adequate disclosure of information, their efforts, consisting of a vague checklist of subjects to be addressed, have not been particularly helpful.

Ironically then, despite the large number of court decisions and varying formulae, there is a lack of clear definition of the scope of required disclosure. With the legal requirements for informed consent unclear, and probably inherently so—given the development of judicially created rules from particular cases with idiosyncratic factual settings—clinicians are probably best advised to fall back on the idea of informed consent for guidance. Sufficient information should be disclosed to provide patients with a genuine opportunity to consider risks and benefits and to participate fully in the selection of appropriate options. Regardless of the formal legal standard, physicians who satisfy their patients' desires for information in this regard are most unlikely to be sued for failure to obtain informed consent. (A method of accomplishing this goal is described in Chapter 8.)

3.4 The Requirement of Consent

The duty of disclosure, or the duty to inform, is the truly distinguishing and innovative aspect of the informed consent doctrine. So much emphasis may be placed on it that one can easily lose sight of the other longstanding duty—that of obtaining consent to treatment.

Consent is not merely the simple matter of the patient's agreement to undergo treatment. Certainly a decision (we prefer this term to consent, since it does not imply whether the patient will agree to a proposed treatment or not) of some sort is essential, but it is only the beginning of the matter. There are two other essential features of a legally valid decision besides assent to or dissent from treatment, to use traditional legal terminology (1, p.233; 64, §49). One is understanding, the other is voluntariness.

Understanding

People are often told things they do not understand, and there is no reason why this simple truth should not operate at least occasionally, perhaps even frequently, in conversations between doctors and patients. In fact, empirical studies suggest that patients frequently fail to understand the information they are told or expected to read. (See Chapter 7.) It has been clear since long before there was any full-scale duty of disclosure that a patient incapable of understanding the nature and consequences of a proposed treatment was deemed incompetent to consent (65,66). But whether an apparently competent patient who fails to understand the disclosure for some other reason—perhaps a failure to attend to certain information or confusion based on conflicting information obtained elsewhere—may render a legally valid consent is uncertain.

In the landmark *Canterbury* opinion, Judge Robinson noted two different ways in which the term informed consent is used:

The doctrine that a consent effective as authority to form [sic; per-form(?)] therapy can arise only from the patient's understanding of alternatives to and risks of the therapy is commonly denominated "in-formed consent." . . . The same appellation is frequently assigned to the doctrine requiring physicians, as a matter of duty to patients to communicate information as to such alternatives and risks (31).

In other words, the term informed consent might denote either the giving of information to a patient or the understanding of information by that patient, or both. The duty of disclosure is fulfilled merely by giving information. The meaning of the word consent as it is used in law generally suggests that there may be an additional requirement of patient understanding. But even after more than a quarter-century of judicial opinions and legislation on informed consent, it remains unclear whether there is any obli-gation on the physician not to render treatment unless the patient understands that information (beyond the basic requirement that the patient not be incompetent), and if so, how that obligation is to be fulfilled.

There are several sources of this uncertainty. First is the use of loose language in judicial opinions. Many courts have failed to distinguish between the physician's giving of information and the patient's receiving of it. Judicial opinions often use words like inform, disclose, tell, know, and understand interchangeably with-out any apparent realization that disclosure of information does not assure the patient's understanding of that information (40,67). This confusion in terminology betrays a deeper uncertainty on the part of the courts as to the true nature of the obligations imposed by the legal requirements of informed consent.

Second, and even more fundamentally, the courts appear un-certain as to the underlying purpose of the legal requirement of informed consent. If the function of the informed consent doctrine is to safeguard the individual's right of choice—however impru-dently exercised—the proper concern is exclusively with the in-formation disclosed by the physician. However, this in no way prohibits the state from adopting means of encouraging patient understanding. If, however, the function of the doctrine is to assure that the decisionmaking process is based on adequate understanding, then the patient's comprehension must also be a focus of judicial concern.

Third, there is uncertainty about the definition of incompetency and the scope of the competency requirement. (See Chapter 5.) Although most informed consent cases do not expressly hold that patients must understand the information disclosed to them before their decision will be considered valid, there is some support for this view in dictum in the case law about incompetency. Justice Cardozo's statement that "[e]very human being of adult years and sound mind has a right to determine what shall be done with his own body" (66) is often echoed in the contemporary informed consent cases (31,38). The judicial statements acknowledging that the decision of a person of unsound mind is legally ineffective do not seem to be directed explicitly toward requiring that patients consistently be tested to determine whether *in fact* they understand the information that is provided to them, and if they do not, to disenfranchising them from making decisions about their health care. Instead the courts seem merely to be establishing a requirement of general competency. However, this conclusion is not at all certain because the courts have not expressly addressed the issue.

A small group of cases more directly suggests that assent to medical care given by a patient who actually has not understood disclosed information is not valid authorization for treatment. In each of these cases the patient claimed that he was under the influence of some therapeutically administered sedative medication that compromised his cognitive faculties. The courts have held that if it can be established that the sedative was administered and that the patient was thereby disabled from understanding information, the patient's authorization of care is not legally valid (8,68,69). However, there is disagreement as to whether the burden is on the plaintiff to establish lack of understanding, or whether the fiduciary nature of the doctor-patient relationship requires the physician to attempt to ascertain the patient's level of understanding and to refrain from proceeding with treatment when comprehension is compromised.

A final source of support for the view that the physician has an obligation to ascertain the patient's level of understanding resides in the meaning of the word consent as it is used in the law generally.

According to the influential treatise on tort law by Harper and James, consent indicates an "assent" given by one who is capable of expressing a rational will (1,pp.234–235). Similarly, the Restatement of Torts indicates that, to be effective, consent must be given by one who has the capacity to consent, which means that "he is capable of appreciating the nature, extent and probable consequences of the conduct consented to" (4,§892A & comment b).

Thus—although there is considerable uncertainty—even if a patient is competent and has been provided adequate information, these facts alone may not render his subsequent decision about medical care legally valid. It may be that the duty of disclosure or the duty to obtain consent, or both, imply a corollary duty on the part of the physician to ascertain that the patient substantially understands the information. Whether or not the law requires understanding, it still seems an integral component of the idea of informed consent. Regardless of the extent of disclosure, patients cannot participate meaningfully in decision making without an understanding of the facts. Physicians dedicated to the principles underlying the law of informed consent should take steps to insure patient understanding even in the absence of a legal requirement.

Voluntariness

There is no doubt that a patient's decision about treatment is not legally effective if the patient has not given it voluntarily. The Restatement of Torts tersely states in this regard that "consent is not effective if it is given under duress" (4,§892B[3]). To state the rule is far simpler than to apply it. There has been virtually no litigation in this context concerning what constitutes duress or, as we prefer to term it, illegitimate pressure. However, since the concept of voluntariness plays a role in a number of other areas of law, some analogical guidance can be derived from them.

Certainly a decision obtained by the use of physical force or the threatened or attempted use of force is highly suspect in its legal and ethical validity. There are circumstances in which patients may be forcibly treated against their will, but (as we discuss in the next two chapters) such situations constitute exceptions to the requirement of informed consent, rather than valid instances of obtaining it. Actual force is clear-cut but likely to be rare in practice.

More troublesome are a variety of verbal pressures that may be imposed on patients, compromising the degree to which they are able freely to consent to or refuse treatment. Human interaction can never be free of pressures that one person consciously or unconsciously places on another. Many pressures are inherent in such interaction and constitute a normal and often desirable part of relationships. Such pressures are often intended to and do in fact influence the behavior of the person toward whom they are directed—for example, when a physician strongly recommends a particular form of treatment. These pressures form a necessary component of socialization and education.

All human behavior involves such pressures, but sometimes they affect behavior so extremely as to deprive it of some of the legal consequences it might otherwise have had. For example, wills are voided if the testator was subjected to undue influence (70, §§5.7, 15.11), criminal confessions are voided if coerced (71), and contracts entered into under duress are voidable (72,§175). So too with consent to medical care. While it is difficult to specify exhaustively the kinds of conduct that will render consent invalid, there can be no doubt as to the general rule (4,§892B[3]).

One aspect of the legitimacy of a decision based on pressure from another person is the legitimacy of the pressure itself. For example, suppose the pressure consisted of a threat that the physician or a family member would whip the patient into agreement. A decision made in response to this pressure could not be considered legitimate because neither the physician nor the family member had the legal (or ethical) right to make such a threat.

Alternatively, where the nature of a pressure is not inherently illegitimate, it may become illegitimate because of its source. The doctrine of informed consent is intended to regulate primarily, if not entirely, the relationship between physicians (or more broadly conceived, health care providers) and patients, not that between other private parties and patients. Thus, there is a significant difference between a situation in which a physician threatens to break off relations with a patient if the recommended surgery is not agreed to, and a situation in which a spouse issues the same threat. The physician's legal (and ethical) right to carry out this threat is seriously limited. If the patient agrees to surgery as a result of this pressure from the physician, the result ought to be different than if the threat is made by a spouse. In the case of the spouse's threat, the patient's choice to undergo surgery is a valid one, in part because of the legitimacy of the pressure placed on him and in part because of the source of the pressure. From a legal perspective, as long as the spouse's threat is legitimate, the patient's choice based in whole or in part on that threat should not be overturned.

In any event, even if the private party administering pressure to a patient has acted illegitimately or unethically, the patient should not necessarily have recourse against a health care provider who administers treatment on the basis of the patient's pressured decision. Health care providers have committed a wrong against the patient only if they have been a party to the private coercion. A physician who enlists a private party to pressure a patient or who collaborates with a private party in pressuring a patient is not free from wrongdoing. More difficult is the case of a physician who knows of a private source of coercion, but does not enlist, cooperate with, or encourage it. Such situations may make some physicians uncomfortable in administering treatment and equally uncomfortable about withholding treatment or intervening in family disputes.

Voluntariness is a critical, though ill-defined, concept. To date, it stands almost alone among issues raised by informed consent in the paucity of analytic thinking being directed to it. While courts have enthusiastically endorsed the dictum that to be effective informed consent must be freely given, they have shied away from the onerous task of giving content and meaning to this concept. This task will become more, rather than less, difficult in the years to come as physicians are increasingly called on to take into consideration the costs and benefits of alternative therapeutic courses when making recommendations to patients.

References

1. Harper FV, James F: *The Law of Torts*. Boston, Little Brown, 1956.
2. I. de S. et ux. v W. de S., in Keeton K, Keeton RE, *Cases and Materials on Torts*. St. Paul, West, 1977.
3. Keeton WP, Dobbs DB, Keeton RE, Owen DG: *Prosser and Keeton on the Law of Torts*. 5th ed. St. Paul, West, 1984.

4. American Law Institute: *Restatement (Second) of the Law of Torts*. St. Paul, American Law Institute Publishers, 1965.

5. Tribe LH: *American Constitutional Law*. Mineola, NY, Foundation Press, 1978.

6. Slater v. Baker & Stapleton, 95 Eng. Rep. 860 (K.B. 1767).

7. Perry v. Hodgson, 140 S.E. 396 (Ga. 1927).

8. Demers v. Gerety, 515 P.2d 645 (N.M. Ct. App. 1973).

9. Rolater v. Strain, 137 Pac. 96 (Okla. 1913).

10. Dicenzo v. Berg, 16 A.2d 15 (Pa. 1940).

11. Markart v. Zeimer, 227 Pac. 683 (Cal. Ct. App. 1924).

12. Meek v. City of Loveland, 276 Pac. 30 (Colo. 1929).

13. Corn v. French, 289 P.2d 173 (Nev. 1955).

14. Kinkead EB: *Commentaries on the Law of Torts: A Philosophic Discussion of the General Principles Underlying Civil Wrongs Ex Delicto*. San Francisco, Bancroft Whitney, 1903.

15. Wall v. Brim, 138 F.2d 478 (5th Cir. 1943).

16. Hunt v. Bradshaw, 88 S.E.2d 762 (N.C. 1955).

17. Waynick v. Reardon, 72 S.E.2d 4 (N.C. 1952).

18. Paulsen v. Gundersen, 260 N.W. 448 (Wis. 1935).

19. State ex rel. Janney v. Housekeeper, 16 Atl. 382 (Md. 1889).

20. Nolan v. Kechijian, 64 A.2d 866 (R.I. 1949).

21. Salgo v. Leland Stanford Jr. Univ. Bd. of Trustees, 317 P.2d 170 (Cal. Ct. App. 1957).

22. Hunter v. Burroughs, 96 S.E. 360 (Va. 1918).

23. Kenny v. Lockwood, [1932] 1 D.L.R. 507 (Ont. Ct. App. 1931).

24. Bang v. Chas. T. Miller Hosp., 88 N.W.2d 186 (Minn. 1958).

25. Hall v. United States, 136 F. Supp. 187 (W.D. La. 1955).

26. Woods v. Pommerening, 271 P.2d 705 (Wash. 1954).

27. Ferrara v. Galluchio, 152 N.E.2d 249 (N.Y. 1958).

28. Katz J: Informed consent—a fairy tale? law's vision. *University of Pittsburgh Law Review* 39:137–174, 1977.

29. Natanson v. Kline, 350 P.2d 1093 (Kan. 1960).

30. Mitchell v. Robinson, 334 S.W.2d 11 (Mo. 1960).

31. Canterbury v. Spence, 464 F.2d 772 (D.C. Cir. 1972).

32. Louisell DW, Williams H: *Medical Malpractice*. Vol. 1. New York, Matthew Bender, 1985.

33. Meisel A: The expansion of liability for medical accidents: from negligence to strict liability by way of informed consent. *Nebraska Law Review* 56:51–152, 1977.

34. Bly v. Rhoads, 222 S.E.2d 783 (Va. 1976).

35. Belli MM: An ancient therapy still applied: the silent medical treatment. *Villanova Law Review* 1:250–289, 1956.

36. Waltz JR: The rise and fall of the locality rule in medical malpractice litigation. *De Paul Law Review* 18:408–420, 1969.

37. Meisel A, Kabnick LD: Informed consent to medical treatment: an analysis of recent legislation. *University of Pittsburgh Law Review* 41:407–564, 1980.

38. Cobbs v. Grant, 502 P.2d 1 (Cal. 1972).

39. Wilkinson v. Vesey, 295 A.2d 676 (R.I. 1972).

40. Cooper v. Roberts, 286 A.2d 647 (Pa. Super. 1971).

41. Waltz JR, Scheuneman TW: Informed consent to therapy. *Northwestern University Law Review* 64:628–650, 1970.

42. President's Commission for the Study of Ethical Problems in Medicine and Biomedical and Behavioral Research: *Making Health Care Decisions: The Ethical and Legal Implications of Informed Consent in the Patient-Practitioner Relationship.* Vol. 3, Appendices. Washington, D.C., U.S. Government Printing Office, 1982. (Appendix L: highlights of state law.)

43. Katz J: *The Silent World of Doctor and Patient.* New York, Free Press, 1984, passim.

44. Lidz CW, Meisel A: Informed consent and the structure of medical care, in President's Commission for the Study of Ethical Problems in Medicine and Biomedical and Behavioral Research, *Making Health Care Decisions: The Ethical and Legal Implications of Informed Consent in the Patient-Practitioner Relationship.* Vol. 2, Appendices. Washington, D.C., U.S. Government Printing Office, 1982.

45. Lidz CW, Meisel A, Zerubavel E, et al.: *Informed Consent: A Study of Decisionmaking in Psychiatry.* New York, Guilford, 1984.

46. McPherson v. Ellis, 305 N.C. 730, 287 S.E.2d 892 (1982), overruled by N.C. Gen. Stat. § 90–21.13 (1981).

47. Weyandt CJ: Valid consent to medical treatment: need the patient know? *Duquesne University Law Review* 4:450–462, 1965–1966.

48. Miller LJ: Informed consent. *JAMA* 244:2100–2103, 2347–2350, 2556–2559, 2661–2662, 1980.

49. Helling v. Carey, 519 P.2d 981 (Wash. 1974).

50. The T. J. Hooper, 60 F.2d 737 (2d Cir. 1932).

51. LeBlang TR: Informed consent—duty and causation: a survey of current developments. *The Forum* 2:280–289, 1983.

52. E.g., Wash. Rev. Code Ann. § 7.70.050(3)(a) (Supp. 1985).

53. E.g., Ohio Rev. Code Ann. § 2317.54(A) (Page 1981).

54. Gray v. Grunnagle, 223 A.2d 663, 674 (Pa. 1966).

55. MacDonald v. Ortho Pharmaceutical Corp., 475 N.E.2d 65 (Mass. 1985).

56. Unthank v. United States, 732 F.2d 1517 (10th Cir. 1984).

57. Petty v. United States, 740 F.2d 1428 (8th Cir. 1984).

58. Archer v. Galbraith, 567 P.2d 1155 (Wash. App. 1977).

59. Tex. Rev. Civ. Stat. Ann. Art. 4590i, §§ 6.03(a), 6.04(a),(d) (Vernon Cum. Supp. 1985).

60. Haw. Rev. Stat. § 671–3(b) (Supp. 1984).

61. Stillman RM, Cohen D, Mitchell WG, et al.: ICBM—A solution to the problem of informed consent. *Journal of Clinical Engineering*, 2:127–132, 1977.

62. Logan v. Greenwich Hosp. Assoc., 465 A.2d 294 (Conn. 1983).

63. Annotation: Medical malpractice: liability for failure of physician to inform patient of alternative modes of diagnosis or treatment. *American Law Reports 3d* 38:901–915, 1985.

64. American Law Institute: *Restatement of the Law of Torts.* St. Paul, American Law Institute Publishers, 1934.

65. Pratt v. Davis, 118 Ill. App. 161 (1905), aff'd 79 N.E. 562 (Ill. 1906).

66. Schloendorff v. Society of New York Hospital, 105 N.E. 92 (N.Y. 1914).

67. Dunham v. Wright, 423 F.2d 940, 944 (3d Cir. 1970).

68. Gravis v. Physicians and Surgeons Hosp., 427 S.W.2d 310 (Tex. 1968).

69. Grannum v. Berard, 422 P.2d 812 (Wash. 1967).

70. Page WH: *Wills*. (Bowe WJ, Parker DH, eds.) Cincinnati, W. H. Anderson, 1960.

71. Spano v. New York, 360 U.S. 315 (1959).

72. American Law Institute: *Restatement (Second) of the Law of Contracts*. St. Paul, American Law Institute Publishers, 1981.

4

Exceptions to the Legal Requirements: Emergency, Waiver, and Therapeutic Privilege

In the preceding chapter we spoke of the requirement for informed consent in absolute terms, as something that was an invariable component of medical decision making. Over the years, courts have come to recognize that there are a number of situations in which physicians are permitted to render treatment without patients' informed consent. Even under the earlier simple consent re quirement, consent to treatment was not required in all situations.

The law does not require that informed consent be obtained when doing so would seriously jeopardize the well-being of a patient, that is, when health values take precedence over the value of individual choice. There are four different kinds of situations in which disclosure and the obtaining of consent could be detrimental to the patient: (1) in an emergency; (2) when the patient waives, or gives up, the right to be informed and/or to consent; (3) when the disclosure itself would harm the patient; and (4) when a patient is incompetent. (Incompetency is addressed in Chapter 5.) Informed consent may also be dispensed with in a fifth set of cases, those of legally required treatment, in which the harm from requiring informed consent is not so much to the patient but to other important societal interests (e.g., civil commitment of the dangerous mentally ill—see Chapter 10).

Each exception contains the potential for undermining the values sought to be implemented by the informed consent doctrine—self-determination and rational decision making. Exceptions that are too broadly defined and applied are a threat to these values. On the other hand, these exceptions are an important vehicle for the interjection into the decisionmaking process of another set of values, those involving the societal interest in the health of the individual. When judiciously defined and applied, the exceptions accord health values their due. However, the exceptions can be and sometimes have been defined so broadly as to dilute, if not dissolve, the fundamental duties imposed by the doctrine and to undermine its essential purpose of assuring patient participation in medical decision making (1).

Since the informed consent requirement imposes not a single duty but two—making disclosure and obtaining consent—exceptions are more complicated than they were under the simple consent requirement. In fact, there is a threshold question that needs to be addressed—namely, exceptions to what? Since there are two duties, it is possible that circumstances will justify a physician's noncompliance with one duty but not the other. That is, in some circumstances a physician may be required to obtain consent but not make disclosure, or vice versa. In other situations, the circumstances may justify omitting both duties.

The ambiguity we described in the last chapter haunts us in considering judicial definitions of the exceptions. Definitions provided in court decisions are often vague and contradictory, even within the same opinion. Therefore, this section anticipates future developments in the law as much as it reflects previous decisions.

4.1 The Emergency Exception

As a general rule, in an emergency a doctor may render treatment without the patient's consent; consent is said to be implied. The rationale for this rule is that since reasonable persons would consent to treatment in an emergency if they were able to do so, it is presumed that any particular patient would consent under the same circumstances (2,§18).

The definition of the term emergency is not clear-cut, though admittedly there is an intuitive or common-sense notion of what it means in a medical context. Many courts have refrained from attempting to define an emergency while still finding one to exist. When they provide any definitions at all, they reflect the various points on a definitional spectrum. At one extreme, an emergency has been said to exist when there was an immediate, serious, and definite threat to life or limb (3). This sort of standard establishes a very high threshold for finding that an emergency exists. Other courts have been far more lenient in recognizing the existence of an emergency. For instance, an emergency has been found to exist sufficient to excuse the failure to obtain consent merely when "suffering or pain [would] be alleviated" by treatment (4).

What should the definition of an emergency be for the purpose of determining when informed consent should be suspended? The answer to this question must take into consideration the extent to which the abandonment or relaxation of informed consent requirements undermines the values the doctrine promotes and the extent to which it promotes the competing value of health.

If informed consent is suspended in an emergency, it should be because the time it would take to make disclosure and obtain patients' decisions would work to the disadvantage of some compelling interest of patients. Thus, the urgency of the need for medical care is a prime determinant of whether a particular situation should be classified as an emergency. How urgent a situation is depends primarily upon the consequences to the patient of delay in the rendition of treatment or failure to render any treatment at all.

The possible consequences of delayed or withheld treatment range from an extreme of death at one end of the spectrum to no consequences at the other. The intermediate consequences vary in nature, degree, and duration. They may involve physical harm, emotional harm, economic harm, or some combination of the three. The harm may be to the patient or to other persons. For instance, in the case of a highly contagious disease, the harm posed is clearly to others as well as to the patient. The psychological harm from delay could conceivably affect members of the patient's family, as could the economic consequences. The degree of harm involved could range from serious to slight, and the duration of harm may vary from momentary to permanent.

If a patient's condition is such that the time necessary for disclosure and consent would be so great that health or life would be seriously jeopardized (e.g., choking, or myocardial infarction), none of the interests promoted by the informed consent doctrine are served. Equally important, to insist upon compliance with informed consent requirements where it would cause grave harm to patients would prevent medical professionals from exercising their skills in compliance with their ethical obligation to provide care for the ill.

Effect of Invoking the Emergency Exception

Because the disclosure obligation is the most time-consuming part of the informed consent requirement (except in the simplest of cases) and is therefore most likely to cause detrimental delay, the emergency exception should ordinarily suspend disclosure.

The applicability of the exception is not as clear, however, in the case of the consent requirement. It is easy to imagine situations so urgent that full disclosure would be counterproductive but not so urgent that consent, possibly following a highly abbreviated disclosure, could not be obtained. For example, a patient who has suffered a severed finger in an accident and who is conscious when brought to the hospital should be asked whether the doctors should attempt to regraft it, and the decision usually should be honored. Minimal disclosure would seem to make sense in such a situation, at least to the extent that the patient might want to know about probability of success and whether the consequences of failure were grave or minimal. Of course, as stated above, where time is of such essence that there will be a grave threat to the patient's life or health if the time is taken to obtain consent, the consent requirement should be suspended too.

4.2 Waiver

Another exception to the requirements of informed consent is known as waiver. A very small number of cases (5–8) and some statutes (9,10) acknowledge that patients may waive their right to give an informed consent to treatment. The statutes and the cases to date, however, do little more than recognize the existence of waiver, leaving some important problems of definition and application unexplicated.

Nonetheless, reasoning by analogy from other areas of the law in which waiver of individual rights has been in issue leads to a fairly certain conclusion as to what constitutes a valid waiver of informed consent. For at least four decades the Supreme Court has defined a waiver as a voluntary and intentional relinquishment of a known right, a definition with substantial common-law precedent (11). This provides a useful starting point.

The Elements of Waiver

In order for patients to waive their right to render informed consent, they must know that they have that right. That is, they must know that (1) physicians have a duty to disclose information to them about treatment, (2) they have a legal right to make decisions about treatment, (3) physicians cannot render treatment without their consent, and (4) the right of decision includes a right to consent to or refuse treatment. Unless a particular patient is far more knowledgeable than most, he or she is unlikely to know all this without being told by the physician. Yet if an obligation were imposed upon physicians to explain patients' rights not to have information disclosed, there is a risk that patients might infer that they ought not to want information or that the physician does not want it disclosed, when as a matter of law patients are entitled to it.

Thus, there should be no absolute obligation to inform patients of their right to waive, but a conditional obligation ought to arise if patients express a desire not to participate in the decisionmaking process. They may do this either by indicating that they do not want information, or that they do not want to decide, or both. Statements like, "Please don't tell me about that, it will only upset me" (the functional equivalent of relinquishment of the right to be informed), or "Doctor, you decide what's best for me, I don't know" (the functional equivalent of relinquishment of the right to decide), should activate the duty to tell patients that they have a right to the information and a right to decide, but also a right to waive. One way of putting this might be for the physician to say, for example, "I'd be glad to stop here if you like, but I want you to know that the final decision about treatment is yours, if you choose to make it, and you have the right to hear as much information as you need to make a decision."

When patients demonstrate a desire to relinquish their rights, physicians should be obligated to ascertain whether they know that they are relinquishing a right, not merely a grace bestowed on them by physicians. There is a very fine line between cases in which patients express desires not to participate and cases in which physicians subtly suggest that they do not care to have patients participate. This fact is a major flaw in suggestions that doctors, in lieu of an affirmative duty of disclosure, inform patients generally that all procedures carry risks and then shift the burden to patients to ask for additional information (12–14).

The Issue of Voluntariness

Well-accepted notions of waiver emphasize that it must be freely and voluntarily given in order to be valid. The issue of voluntariness in the context of waiver of informed consent is closely related to, and as unclear as, the same issue in the context of consent itself. In other words, both consent and waiver of informed consent are subtypes of the same general category, which we might call making a decision. In the case of consent (or informed consent), patients decide about treatment; in the case of waiver, patients decide either that they do not want information, or to let someone else decide, or both. Both situations affect patients' decisional rights. Thus, as in consent to treatment, a waiver would certainly not be voluntary if physical force were applied by physicians to compel patients' relinquishment of their rights. Of course, it would be highly unusual for such a situation to occur. A more plausible situation might involve a material misrepresentation of fact to patients—for example, telling them that they have no right to information, or no right to decide—which might be viewed as making any subsequent relinquishment involuntary. (In other words, patients do not relinquish a *known* right under such circumstances.)

If misrepresentation of facts about the nature of the treatment (such as risks, benefits, or alternatives) induces patients to relinquish their rights, it should also be viewed as rendering waiver involuntary. For example, a physician, not wishing to disclose information to patients, and wishing to be absolved of the disclosure duty by obtaining a patient's waiver, might inform a patient that the contemplated procedures are very simple and the patient should not be concerned about them, when in fact they are complicated and risky (15).

The Waiver Exception in Perspective

Because the doctrine of informed consent is designed to permit patients to make decisions and to provide them with information so that they may make them rationally, an exception that denies them this information seems to undermine these goals. However, assuring that decision making is rational is not the sole or ultimate goal of the doctrine of informed consent. Rather, the primary objective of the doctrine is to promote individual self-determination. *Permitting* patients to make such decisions is one way of fostering self-determination. On the other hand, *compelling* them to receive information they do not want or make decisions they do not wish to make is a denial of the right of self-determination, even though in this case the consequence is that patients will *not* participate fully (or at all) in decision making. Thus, a waiver, properly given, is in keeping with the values sought to be promoted by informed consent because the patient remains the ultimate decision maker.

Patients should be able to waive either or both of the duties imposed upon physicians. They should be able to give up the right to information without relinquishing the right to decide, or vice versa. They might determine that they wish neither to be informed nor to decide.

Waiver permits patients to be protected from any harmful impact *they* believe disclosure might have upon them or from the possible anxiety that may accompany the decisionmaking process. Patients here, not doctors, determine that disclosure or decision making will be harmful. The case is otherwise for therapeutic privilege.

4.3 Therapeutic Privilege

Physicians may in appropriate circumstances withhold information they would otherwise be obliged to disclose if disclosure would be harmful to a patient. Of all the exceptions to the informed consent doctrine this is the best known and most discussed, despite the fact that the outcome of very few cases turns on its application.

Although the contours of therapeutic privilege are uncertain, its general purpose is clear: to "free physicians from a legal requirement which would force them to violate their 'primary duty' to do what is beneficial for the patient" (16). Others have said that the privilege permits doctors to uphold their professional, ethical obligation to "do no harm" (17). The source of this obligation in the informed consent context is unclear, and its existence in law appears mostly in dictum (18). In practice, it is likely that the privilege serves to legitimate the natural aversion of physicians to disclosing information to patients (19–21). Thus, if the scope of the privilege is not severely circumscribed, it contains the potential to swallow the general obligation of disclosure. If the harm to patients from disclosure is viewed broadly, as it occasionally has been by the courts (22), to include the risk that patients may choose to reject medical care, the privilege would in effect permit physicians to substitute their judgment for patients' in every instance of medical decision making. Therefore, it should be made clear that "[t]he privilege does not accept the paternalistic notion that the physician may remain silent simply because divulgence might prompt the patient to forego therapy the physician feels the patient really needs" (23). The boundaries of the privilege ought to be defined in terms of the primary functions of the informed consent doctrine, rather than by reference to the harm that may be done to the patient by disclosure. Thus, if the doctrine exists primarily to promote patient participation in medical decision making and to promote rational decision making, information should only be permitted to be withheld if its disclosure would thwart one of these objectives.

Judicial Formulations

In the landmark informed consent case of *Canterbury* v. *Spence*, the court seemed to have adopted this approach when it stated that information about the possible untoward consequences of the treatment may be withheld from patients because "[i]t is recognized that patients occasionally become so ill or emotionally distraught on disclosure as to foreclose a rational decision" (23). That is, information may be withheld when its disclosure would so upset patients that they would be unable to engage in decision making in a rational way or at all.

Other courts have not confined themselves to so restrictive a definition of the privilege. One of the few cases whose result actually turned on the therapeutic privilege, *Nishi* v. *Hartwell*, formulated it so as to permit physicians extensive leeway in withholding information. The court stated that because

> the doctrine [of informed consent] recognizes that the primary duty of a physician is to do what is best for his patient . . . a physician may withhold disclosure of information regarding any untoward consequences of a treatment where full disclosure will be detrimental to the patient's total care and best interest (24).

At another point, the court suggested that information might be properly withheld from the patient if its disclosure "might induce an adverse psychosomatic reaction in a patient highly apprehensive of his condition." Patients might conceivably have mild, transitory "psychosomatic reactions" (e.g., anxiety reactions characterized by increased pulse, rapid breathing, flushing, etc.) to the disclosure of risk information, yet it is questionable whether these would interfere with their decisionmaking ability. Such a standard is not functionally related to patients' abilities to participate in decision making. Moreover, it emphasizes the value of patients' health almost to the exclusion of the right to choose.

In addition to its stringent formulation of the privilege, the *Canterbury* case also contains language suggesting that there are less restrictive circumstances in which it should properly apply. In fact, the court's most general statement is that the privilege applies "when risk disclosure poses such a threat of detriment to the patient as to become unfeasible or contraindicated from a medical point of view" (23). However, the court took pains to explain that it did not intend that the privilege be framed so broadly

> that the physician may remain silent simply because divulgence might prompt the patient to forego therapy the physician feels the patient really needs. That attitude presumes instability or perversity for even

the normal patient, and runs counter to the foundation principle that the patient should and ordinarily can make the choice for himself (23).

The privilege is to operate only "where the patient's reaction to risk information, as reasonabl[y] foreseen by the physician, is menacing." Yet, the court did not limit the operation of the privilege merely to those situations in which disclosure would so upset the patient as to preclude participation in decisionmaking. It would also permit the privilege to operate when risk disclosure would "complicate or hinder the treatment" or "pose psychological damage to the patient."

The discussion of the privilege in *Canterbury* is confused by the use of some language suggesting a strict formulation and other language suggesting a looser formulation. Because of these conflicting formulations, the case nicely exemplifies the disparate values sought to be reconciled by the general rule of informed consent and the exception for therapeutic reasons. Although disclosure of treatment information and patient decision making are important, if not compelling, values, they should not be pursued so singlemindedly that they become self-defeating. When disclosure clearly threatens to impede rather than promote patient decision making, consideration must be given to dispensing with it. In fact, there is some authority suggesting that disclosure *must* be suspended when it poses an unreasonable threat of harm to patients (25–27).

When properly invoked, the therapeutic privilege does not necessarily contemplate complete nondisclosure. The *Canterbury* formulation of the privilege indicates that it is primarily, if not exclusively, information about the risks of treatment that may be withheld, although if the disclosure of information about the purpose, benefits, or alternatives would interfere substantially with patients' decisionmaking capacity, it is reasonable to assume that such disclosure should be also dispensed with or abbreviated.

Whether or not the privilege contemplates that the duties of both disclosure and consent are suspended is not clear. Since the discussion of the privilege in *Canterbury* is framed primarily in terms of relieving physicians of the duty to disclose risk information, the implication is that physicians are still obligated to disclose all other relevant information and to obtain consent as well. In fact, it is difficult to see how giving consent to treatment would ever seriously "menace" (23) a patient's physical or psychological well-being. Yet the court in *Canterbury* ends its discussion of the therapeutic privilege with the suggestion that when the privilege is invoked, disclosure should be made to a close relative "with a view to securing consent to the proposed treatment" (23). Although the court does not clearly address the issue, a fair reading is that the consent of the relative is to be obtained in lieu of the patient's consent and not in addition to it (28). *Nishi* explicitly states, on the other hand, that disclosure need not have been made to the patient's wife because only the patient's own consent, and not his wife's, was necessary to authorize treatment (24). We believe that the duty to obtain consent should not be abrogated by the invocation of the therapeutic privilege. To do so would unnecessarily compromise patients' right to decide, without any corresponding gain to their health.

The Therapeutic Privilege in Perspective

To the extent that it merely dispenses with the disclosure of risk information while continuing to require physicians to disclose all other information and to obtain patients' consent to treatment, the privilege still permits patients a measure of decisional authority. If the need for patients' consent is dispensed with, but the consent of close relatives is still required, some protection is provided against excessive medical zeal, and some room is made for the interjection of nonmedical values into the decisionmaking process. However, such nonmedical values will not be those of patients, unless relatives inadvertently or intentionally express patients' views instead of their own.

As stated above, a stringently formulated privilege is most consistent with the individualistic values sought to be promoted by the informed consent doctrine. The effect of even a stringently formulated privilege is easily undercut by rules related to its application. Whether a lay or professional standard is applied to determine whether disclosure would have harmed a patient, whether expert testimony other than that of the defendant is necessary to show that a patient would have been harmed by full disclosure, and whether the burden of proof is on physicians or patients—all these factors will critically affect how the balance is struck between individualism and health.

Some commentators believe that the therapeutic privilege poses so great a danger to self-determination in medical decision making that its abolition might seriously be considered. To do so would not be as revolutionary as it might seem at first, because of the overlap between the therapeutic privilege and two of the other exceptions: waiver and incompetency. The waiver exception might serve as sufficient means of reconciling patients' right to and need for information with the obligation of physicians to do no harm. To reduce the risk of upsetting patients, while avoiding the substantially reduced disclosure consequent to the application of the therapeutic privilege, physicians might tell patients something like the following: "There is some information about your treatment that you may wish to know, and I will tell you about it if you like. There's a chance that this information may upset you, and if you'd rather that I not go into detail, please say so. And if you'd like, I'll discuss it with your spouse [or other family member] instead." Such a statement shifts the responsibility for halting harmful disclosure to patients, keeping them, not their physicians, in control of their right of self-determination.

As currently conceived, the therapeutic privilege overlooks the possibility that if patients were asked to make a prospective determination, they might decide that they prefer to be harmed by being informed than be harmed by having to make choices in the dark of nondisclosure. In contrast, waiver— operating in the manner previously described—permits patients to make this very determination. It is possible that even the limited disclosure that "this information may upset you" will harm patients (29), though this is not likely. But to require this minimal preparatory disclosure does not seem an unreasonable compromise between the competing interests of patients' rights to disclosure and consent and the interest (and physicians' ethical obligation) to do no harm.

In some cases in which the therapeutic privilege might be invoked there is also room for the operation of the incompetency exception, depending in part on how that exception is defined. This is especially so when a physician has experience with a particular patient and can more reasonably predict how the patient will react to frightening information (20). Patients whose emotional states are so fragile that risk disclosure might seriously harm them or prevent them from participating rationally in decision making might be considered incompetent, depending on what standard for determining incompetency is applied. (See Chapter 5 for a full discussion of the incompetency exception.)

The abolition of the therapeutic privilege might have another salutary effect on the physician-patient relationship. Although physicians may not actually know of the privilege by name, they probably have a general understanding that the law permits them to withhold information that might harm patients. The therapeutic privilege has been extensively written about in medical journals, and it is reasonable to assume that physicians have at least a passing acquaintance with the concept. There is equally good reason to believe that most people suspect that physicians withhold information from patients, thus undermining the trust that is thought to be highly desirable in promoting good therapeutic results (12). The affirmative act of abolishing the privilege might be viewed as a withdrawal of the legitimation of physicians' natural reticence to disclose information.

At the present time, there is insufficient empirical evidence to validate the basis for the therapeutic privilege—that is, that patients can be harmed by disclosure of information *per se*. Unusual case examples might be imagined (e.g., a patient with an unstable cardiac arrhythmia being asked to consent to its treatment, the explanation of which might heighten anxiety and thus increase the risk of sudden death), but even if the privilege were retained to take them into account, there is still no valid reason to preserve a privilege that is so loosely defined. If there is any room at all for it, it must be framed narrowly in terms of interference with patients' decisionmaking capabilities.

Conclusion

The exceptions of emergency, waiver, and therapeutic privilege play an important role in the theoretical and day-to-day functioning of the legal doctrine of informed consent. The interplay between the values of autonomy and of health has been clearly evident in their formulation and application, and in the continuing controversy that these exceptions—particularly therapeutic privilege—

engender. As intricate and subject to dispute as the issues raised in this chapter are, the fourth major exception to the requirement for informed consent—incompetency—is far more complex and controversial.

References

1. Meisel A: The "exceptions" to the informed consent doctrine: striking a balance between competing values in medical decisionmaking. *Wisconsin Law Review* 1979:413–488.

2. Keeton WP, Dobbs DB, Keeton RE, Owen DG: *Prosser and Keeton on the Law of Torts.* 5th ed. St. Paul, West, 1984.

3. Cunningham v. Yankton Clinic, P.A., 262 N.W.2d 508 (S.D. 1978).

4. Sullivan v. Montgomery, 279 N.Y.S. 575 (City Ct. 1935).

5. Cobbs v. Grant, 502 P.2d 1 (Cal. 1972).

6. Putensen v. Clay Adams, Inc., 12 Cal. App.3d 1062, 1083–84 (1970).

7. Kaimowitz v. Michigan Dep't of Mental Health, 1 Ment. Dis. Law Rprt. 147 (Cir. Ct. Wayne County Mich. 1976).

8. Holt v. Nelson, 523 P.2d 211, 219 (Wash. App. 1974).

9. N.Y. Pub. Health Law § 2805-d(4)(b) (McKinney 1977).

10. Utah Code Ann. § 78-14-5.2(c) (1977).

11. 28 Am. Jur. 2d, *Estoppel and Waiver* § 154, at 836 (1966).

12. Alfidi RJ: Controversy, alternatives, and decisions in complying with the legal doctrine of informed consent. *Radiology* 114:231–234, 1975.

13. Lankton JW, Batchelder BM, Ominsky AJ: Emotional responses to detailed risk disclosure for anesthesia—a prospective randomized study. *Anesthesiology* 46:294–296, 1977.

14. Or. Rev. Stat. § 677.097 (1977).

15. E.g., Paulsen v. Gundersen, 260 N.W. 448 (Wis. 1935).

16. Informed consent: the illusion of patient choice. *Emory Law Journal* 23:503–522, 1974.

17. Lund CC: The doctor, the patient, and the truth. *Tennessee Law Review* 344–348, 1946.

18. Salgo v. Leland Stanford Jr. Univ. Bd. of Trustees, 317 P.2d 170 (Cal. App. 1957).

19. Schneyer TJ: Informed consent and the danger of bias in the formation of medical disclosure practices. *Wisconsin Law Review* 1976:124–170.

20. Meisel A, Roth LH: Toward an informed discussion of informed consent: a review and critique of the empirical studies. *Arizona Law Review* 25:265–346, 1983.

21. Glass ES: Restructuring informed consent: legal therapy for the doctor-patient relationship. *Yale Law Journal* 79:1533–1576, 1970.

22. Barclay v. Campbell, 683 S.W.2d 498, 501 (Tex. Civ. App. 1984).

23. Canterbury v. Spence, 464 F.2d 772 (D.C. Cir. 1972).

24. Nishi v. Hartwell, 473 P.2d 116 (Haw. 1970).
25. Williams v. Menehan, 379 P.2d 292, 294 (Kan. 1963).
26. Ferrara v. Galluchio, 152 N.E.2d 249 (N.Y. 1958).
27. Kraus v. Spielberg, 236 N.Y.S.2d 143 (Sup. Ct. 1962).
28. Cornfeldt v. Tongen, 262 N.W.2d 684, 701 n.14 (Minn. 1977).
29. Blumenfield M, Levy NB, Kaufman D: Do patients want to be told? *N Engl J Med* 299:1128, 1978.

5

Exceptions to the Legal Requirements: Incompetency

It has been recognized since the earliest cases dealing with consent that certain individuals are incompetent to consent to treatment, and that they may be treated without their consent (1,2). The alternative to treatment without the patient's consent would be no treatment at all (3), a result that would make a fetish of consent, for it would mean that those lacking the ability to make medical decisions would be required to forego medical care.

The exception for incompetent patients is closely related to the emergency exception. In fact, many situations involve an overlap of the two exceptions, since many cases of genuine emergency treatment involve unconscious (and thus incompetent) patients. The class of incompetent patients includes more than just those who are unconscious, though, and situations arise involving the treatment of incompetent patients that are not emergencies.

Making medical decisions in cases involving incompetent patients has been an area of great confusion, though the fog may be slowly beginning to lift. The first step in clarifying the matter is to understand that there are a number of different but interrelated issues embedded in the problem of decision making for incompetent patients. These issues need to be sorted out before they can be intelligently addressed.

First, there is the substantive issue of defining the scope of the problem itself, which in this case means defining what is meant by an incompetent patient. Until that is done, the boundaries of the problem have not even been established. This threshold issue, unfortunately, is in a state of great confusion. Although we can go on to talk about the other issues, and in clinical settings can follow a set of procedures for decision making with patients deemed incompetent, we may still be left with a nagging doubt about whether the particular patient actually is incompetent.

Second, a closely related procedural issue is also largely unsettled, or at least there is a large gulf between legal theory and clinical practice. Who is or ought to be empowered to determine whether a patient is incompetent? Taken together, we might characterize these two threshold issues in the incompetency conundrum as: By what standards should a person be declared incompetent and who should make that decision?

Assuming for argument's sake that these issues can be satisfactorily resolved—and in practice they usually are—the remaining issues are largely procedural. Who should decide for the incompetent patient? Must informed consent be obtained from this surrogate? By what standards should the surrogate decide? Should there be any review of such a decision, if so by whom, and utilizing what criteria?

5.1 General versus Specific Incompetency

Strictly speaking, persons are legally incompetent if they are minors or, if adults, they have been determined by a court (adjudicated) to be incompetent. A person who is incompetent suffers certain legal disabilities. Traditionally, an adjudication of incompetency placed an individual under total legal disability, and a guardian was appointed to make all decisions on the individual's behalf. In practice, such incompetency affected primarily financial matters. In recent years, increasing attention has been paid to whether the adjudication of incompetency and appointment of a guardian should render the person incompetent for all purposes. Some states have dealt with this problem through the enactment of statutes, others through judicial decisions, distinguishing between general and specific incompetency. An adjudication of general incompetency continues to render the person incompetent for all purposes. An adjudication of specific incompetency, as the term suggests, renders the person incompetent only for limited purposes, which are indicated in a court order.

Even in jurisdictions without such statutes or judicial precedents, an adjudication of incompetency may still have only limited effect if the court order appointing a guardian is narrowly drafted. For example, the order may appoint a guardian for the delineated purposes of managing the person's financial affairs, consenting to a particular surgical operation, selling a particular piece of property, or making decisions about the person's place of residence (e.g., a nursing home).

In the case of minors, even age does not render a person incompetent for all purposes. In many states, statutes exist permitting older children validly to authorize the administration of certain limited kinds of medical care (e.g., treatment for mental illness, substance abuse, venereal disease, pregnancy), or the common law may permit mature minors validly to consent to medical care (4–6).

5.2 Standards for Determining Incompetency

The threshold problem raised by the incompetency exception is that of defining what is meant by incompetency. There are no well-accepted standards for incompetency (7,8). The courts have spoken in vague generalities and no comprehensive judicial exegesis of the subject has yet appeared. What is important is that the criteria selected for the determination of incompetency ought to promote the values sought to be achieved by the doctrine of informed consent (primarily individual autonomy, secondarily rational decisionmaking), while showing due regard for the preservation or promotion of the patient's health.

Not only are there no well-accepted standards for determining incompetency, but there is also considerable confusion as to the appropriate procedures for making such a determination (see Sections 5.3 and 5.4). Although the courts are always available to make such determinations, it is customary practice in the medical profession for a patient's attending physician to do so. In any event clinicians, of necessity, must provide the first level of screening for incompetency, since the initial decision as to whether or not to accept a patient's decision rests with them. Thus, clinicians require guidance as to what standards courts may look to in judging incompetency.

The determination of incompetency can be approached in several different ways. Each has been utilized, or its appropriateness suggested, in court decisions, statutes, administrative regulations, or scholarly commentary.

Specific Incompetency

The first set of approaches to establishing standards for the determination of incompetency focuses on the behavior of a patient in the context of the medical decisionmaking process. These approaches are referred to as "specific incompetency" because they are concerned with the patient's competency to make a medical decision, rather than with the patient's competency in general.

PRESENCE OF DECISION

One standard for incompetency focuses on the mere presence (or absence) of a patient's decision. That is, the patient who chooses one treatment rather than another, or no treatment at all, could be deemed competent without regard to the manner in which the choice was made and without regard to the nature of the choice itself. On the other hand, a patient who, when asked to decide, does not do so is deemed incompetent. Again, no inquiry is made into the reasons for the patient's failure to decide, if indeed such an exploration could be made. The mere failure to manifest a choice is determinative of the issue.

Although patients who do not manifest a decision should be treated as incompetent, the opposite is not always true. Whether patients who manifest a choice should be automatically considered competent depends upon the weight to be accorded self-determination at the expense of competing values. If the ability merely to manifest a decision is accepted as the standard for competency, persons who have no ability to comprehend what they are deciding about, but object nonetheless, will be able to thwart the administration of treatments, some of which may be highly beneficial and relatively risk-free.

ACTUAL UNDERSTANDING

Competency could also be viewed as corresponding to a patient's understanding of the information required to be disclosed by the informed consent doctrine. A patient who does not know, appreciate, or comprehend the requisite elements of disclosure could be considered incompetent (9). No inquiry would be made into how the patient arrives at the ultimate treatment decision or into the nature of the decision itself.

To be competent, patients would have to understand the factual basis for their decision. Conversely, failing to grasp essential information would render one incompetent. However, in the application of a standard that requires a determination of "understanding" the problem arises that in attempting to gauge understanding, the values of the tester play an insidious, and probably unavoidable role. Not only does the tester's view of what constitutes understanding affect the determination, but the initial selection of the information the patient is to be tested on reflects the importance the tester attaches to that information. Thus, the personal identity and professional allegiance of the tester play an influential role. If the tester is a physician or other clinician, health values may receive great weight.

A further problem with this standard is that large numbers of persons may be found incompetent if a high level of understanding is expected. The level of understanding that a reasonable person could be expected to have should be appropriate, but physicians may have difficulty recognizing just how low this level may be. An actual-understanding test is probably the standard with which laypeople and lawyers are most comfortable.

THE NATURE OF THE DECISIONMAKING PROCESS

A more complex standard for incompetency focuses on the nature of the decisionmaking process employed by a patient. After patients are provided with and presumably understand the requisite information about treatment options, inquiry is made into the manner in which they make their decisions. This standard can be framed to examine two related but distinct issues: whether the patient engages in rational manipulation of available information, and whether the patient appreciates the implications of a decision.

The first question might be addressed by looking at whether the patient applies a utilitarian calculus—weighing the risks against the benefits of treatment; whether the patient has taken into account each of the elements of disclosure (see Section 3.3); or whether delusions, hallucinations, or a thought disorder materially influence the decision. The second factor might be evaluated by examining the weight the patient accords each of the elements of information involved. Or a patient who gives so-called unsound reasons for consenting or refusing might be viewed as incompetent (10). Numerous other variations exist.

This approach to the determination of incompetency honors health values more than tests that merely look to the presence of a decision on the part of the patient, or even the patient's understanding. The basic view is that if a patient is able to make a decision, but unable to make it in the preferred manner, then the decision is somewhat less of a decision and deserves less to be honored. The unstated premise is that there is a greater chance that if the decision is made improperly, reliance on it will be detrimental to the patient's medical well-being. Therefore, by not obligating the physician to honor such a decision, society's interest in advancing health and the profession's interest in ministering to ameliorable illness are promoted. Many, however, are uncomfortable with the degree of discretion this standard lodges in the medical profession—even more than a test of actual understanding.

THE NATURE OF THE DECISION

Rather than focusing on characteristics of the patient or how the patient makes a decision, another alternative is to examine the nature of the decision itself. For example, a patient who chooses no treatment over treatment or one who chooses a risky treatment over a less risky one could be said to be incompetent. One problem with this approach is that it is difficult if not impossible objectively to rank the seriousness of various kinds of hazards. For example, which is the greater hazard, paralysis or blindness? The answer depends on circumstances that vary from situation to situation, ultimately making the resolution highly subjective. Another problem is that a treatment rarely has only one material hazard associated with it. Thus, a patient must weigh combinations of hazards or of hazards and benefits, substantially complicating any sort of ranking. Or a patient whose decision could simply be termed wrong, unreasonable, irrational, and so forth, might be found incompetent.

The most fundamental problem with this approach is that a standard by which the nature of the decision determines whether the patient is incompetent seriously undermines individual autonomy. Such a standard is paternalistic to an extreme. It does not even maintain a pretense of seeking to achieve a balance between competing values, but instead completely eliminates the role of autonomy. Another serious (though less fundamental) problem is that this test is probably biased in favor of decisions by patients to accept treatment (i.e., consent), even when the consent is given by a patient who does not understand any of the information disclosed or is unable to weight the risks and benefits. If the patient consents, the physician's bias in favor of treatment (especially one the physician has taken the time to inform the patient about and presumably recommends) will cause the physician to judge the patient competent merely because the patient has agreed with the favored recommendation (7).

General Incompetency

The foregoing are standards for specific incompetency, in that they examine the patient's conduct in the context of the medical decisionmaking process, though each focuses on a different aspect of the process. Another approach focuses on certain qualities of persons whose competency is in question as persons rather than as patients—that is, as they function outside the medical decisionmaking context rather than within it. For example, an individual whose overall functioning is impaired by permanent conditions such as severe mental retardation or temporary conditions such as alcohol or drug intoxication could be viewed as incompetent (11–19). Other conditions, such as certain psychiatric illnesses or symptoms, might also severely impair an individual's overall functioning. One might even focus on such items as the patient's appearance (20). This approach might be made slightly more specific by looking not at general ability to function but at ability to make decisions in general—as opposed to ability to make medical decisions (21). In some respects the general incompetency standard could be viewed as encompassing the first four tests, because it attempts to infer a person's capacity for participation in medical decision making from his or her overall ability to function rather than determining it in a limited way in the medical context.

The general incompetency standard attempts to predict specific incompetency for medical decision making on the basis of certain characteristics of the patient. Under this standard, it is assumed that if patients are intoxicated, retarded, or psychotic, and disclosure were made, they could not understand, make rational decisions, or participate in a rational way, and so they are not given the opportunity to do so. Thus competency is determined by the patient's *potential* ability to meet one or more of the four standards already described: (1) to evidence a decision, (2) to actually understand the information about the treatment under consideration, (3) to engage in decision making in a rational way, with an appreciation of the potential outcomes, or (4) to make a decision about treatment that is reasonable in itself. The value of the concept of general incompetency is that it alerts the physician to the fact that the patient may be specifically incompetent.

The problems with a general incompetency standard are twofold. First, there may be little correspondence between a determination of general incompetency and a patient's ability to participate in medical decision making, however that ability may be determined. A patient who appears to be generally incompetent may actually be capable of making decisions if a reasonable amount of time and energy are spent in the attempt. Secondly, this standard can only be applied either mechanically or subjectively. A mechanical standard would deem incompetent any individual who could be reasonably characterized as, for example, intoxicated or psychotic. While a mechanical standard has administrative convenience and frees physicians from being second-guessed by juries, it suffers from the serious deficiency of not necessarily being functionally related to actual decisionmaking ability. For example, if all persons with IQs less that 75 were deemed incompetent to make medical decisions by virtue of their IQ, it would be relatively simple to determine who is competent and who is not. However, it is certain that there are persons with IQs greater than 75 who may not be competent to make medical decisions in certain circumstances, such as an intoxicated auto accident victim. Conversely, there are probably some people with IQs less than 75 who are capable of understanding the relevant information, at least about certain medical procedures that may be recommended for them. The only alternative, however, is standardless subjectivity. In either case, it is uncertain whether values of self-determination will be given their proper weight.

A Conjunctive Approach

Although the general incompetency standard may be viewed as an alternative to one of the specific incompetency standards, the two can and should operate in conjunction. The general incompetency standard should be used as a threshold standard for incompetency. That is, ordinarily the duties of disclosure and consent are suspended if the patient is generally incompetent. To take the most extreme example, if a patient is unconscious the doctor need not fulfill the disclosure or the consent requirement. These duties would also be suspended in less extreme situations, such as severe intoxication. In other words, general competency is a threshold that must be surmounted—that is, a condition that must be met—before the doctor is obligated to make disclosure and to obtain consent.

If patients are determined to be generally competent (which they are legally presumed to be), physicians are obligated to attempt disclosure. After an effort to disclose and obtain consent has begun, it may yet become apparent that the patient is specifically incompetent by reference to one or more of the four standards described above: the patient (1) does not manifest a decision, (2) does not understand the disclosure, (3) does not engage in the proper sort of decisionmaking process, or (4) does not arrive at the proper decision.

Thus, the determination of incompetency is a two-step process, having a varied effect upon the obligations imposed by the informed consent doctrine. First, the duty of disclosure and the duty of obtaining consent are suspended only if the patient fails to meet the threshold standard of general incompetency. Second, if the patient is not generally incompetent, specific incompetency will suspend the obligation of obtaining consent, though not necessarily of making disclosure, for it may be only in the process of making disclosure that the patient's specific incompetency becomes apparent.

Precisely which of the four standards of specific incompetency is employed should be a function of the law in a particular jurisdiction. Since the law in many states is so vague as to provide no guidance, however, physicians will often be in the position of selecting the standard themselves. Ideally, providers likely to face questions of competency should arrive in advance at agreement on standards to be employed; this process can involve clinicians, administrators, and legal counsel. In any event, the confusion in this area makes it essential that clinicians have a clear idea in their own minds of what standards they are applying and be able to explicate them if the issue comes to court. Some commentators have suggested that the standard to be employed could vary with the consequences of the patient's decision (22). Others have favored use of a stable set of criteria regardless of the situation, perhaps combining the presence-of-decision, understanding, and process-of-decision-making tests (23).

Whatever the standard, if the patient fails to meet the criteria for competency, the physician's obligation to obtain *consent* from the patient is suspended. The patient's decision (if any is rendered) need not be honored, and the decision as to whether and how the patient is to be treated may be made without his or her further participation, although further legal proceedings, depending on the treatment and the jurisdiction, may be required.

5.3 Who Makes the Determination?

In theory, the determination of incompetency requires the official legal act known as adjudication. An adjudicated incompetent is referred to as *de jure* incompetent. In practice, however, many people who have not been subjected to an adjudication of incompetency are deemed incompetent to manage their financial and/or personal affairs. Such people are called *de facto* incompetent; they are incompetent in fact, but have not by legal procedures been determined to be so.

Consideration of persons who are incompetent to manage their financial affairs sheds light on related problems with medical decision making. In many cases, the absence of wealth and complicated financial problems militates against invoking so formal, cumbersome, and potentially expensive a proceeding as an adjudication of incompetency and the concurrent appointment of a guardian to manage the incompetent's estate. Family members often make less formal arrangements for an incompetent person's financial affairs. For example, if a person is having difficulty remembering to pay utility bills, a relative may take over the job by means of a joint checking account. Or if an elderly person suddenly starts to give away to strangers all of the money needed for living, arrangements can be made with the Social Security Administration to have a relative named representative payee (24), to whom Social Security checks are then sent to be used for the elderly person's living expenses.

An important distinction between the informal mechanisms of de facto incompetency and the more formal appointing of a guardian concerns accountability. Court-appointed guardians must account to the court on a regular basis for the assets of the incompetent that have been entrusted to them. Although legal remedies do exist to call to account a person who has failed to use a de facto incompetent's assets for the benefit of the incompetent, these remedies are expensive and unwieldy. Furthermore, they will not operate at all unless the incompetent or someone else is aware that the incompetent's assets are being misused and is willing to assert the incompetent's rights.

In practice, determinations of incompetency to make medical decisions proceed much the same way as determinations of incompetency to handle financial affairs, despite assertions by some commentators that medical decisions can or should be made for an incompetent patient only by a court-appointed guardian (25, p. 33; 26). Most cases simply do not warrant the invocation of legal proceedings. The issues are not complex and the cost of legal proceedings is great, at least in relation to the simplicity of the issues involved. The delay attendant to seeking an adjudication of incompetency might add substantially to the cost of care if the patient is hospitalized, and might sometimes be injurious to the patient's health (27). Ordinarily, family members make decisions about medical care for *de facto* incompetent persons (we will refer to such a family member as a surrogate) in much the same way that they take over their financial affairs (25, pp. 126–132). Only in a small proportion of cases is an adjudication of incompetency sought: generally when there is no family member to make decisions, when the family member makes a decision that the attending physician believes to be detrimental to the well-being of the patient, when there is intractable conflict among family members over what course to pursue, or when it is unclear whether legal liability (either criminal or civil) might be incurred as a result of the particular kind of decision that needs to be made.

Again in the area of accountability, there is one important distinction between informal medical decision making and the handling of financial affairs. As mentioned earlier with respect to financial affairs, accountability is haphazard at best. In medical decision making, there is a safeguard in that there are other persons concerned with the patient's welfare besides the surrogate. Thus, if the surrogate makes a decision out of improper motives or a decision that will be harmful to the patient, at least some other party will know of it. Although this situation does not guarantee that action will be taken to prevent harm to the patient, there is a greater likelihood of protection than with respect to financial matters.

Because most patients are in fact competent to make medical decisions and because of the legal presumption of competency, if there is to be a more formal inquiry into incompetency, something must trigger it. Often this trigger will be the fact that the patient refuses a recommended treatment. (It should be noted that refusal of treatment is not the same as a lack of capacity to decide about treatment.) The initiation of the inquiry will ordinarily be in the clinical setting, but final resolution of the matter of the patient's incompetency may or may not occur there.

It has not been settled whether, for practical purposes, the final determination of incompetency must be made by a court or whether it may be made in the clinical setting without judicial participation. There is a long tradition in medical practice of physicians relying upon family members to make decisions on behalf of patients unable to do so themselves. The practice of obtaining consent from a family member, warns Capron, "is so well known in society at large that any individual who finds the prospect particularly odious has ample warning to make other arrangements better suited to protecting his own ends or interests" (28).

In other words, determinations that a patient is incompetent are frequently— indeed, overwhelmingly—made by physicians at a low level of visibility. Such determinations have been made not only routinely, but also largely without a conscious awareness on the part of the participants of what they were doing. To call such a process a determination is to accord it far too much formality. Such a determination is usually only an implicit byproduct of the physician's more overt decision to engage in medical decision making not with the patient but with the family.

Doubt about the legitimacy of this process lingers because of a number of factors. First, all states have statutory procedures for the determination of incompetency through the judicial process (29). Courts might determine that these statutes authorize the sole legally valid means for making such a determination. Second, there are reported cases in many, if not all, jurisdictions in which physicians, or hospital administrators acting at their behest, have sought an adjudication of incompetency. Only rarely has a court suggested that resort to the judicial process for such a determination was unwarranted (30). The very fact that courts do make such adjudications indicates that the professional custom is not entirely clear-cut. There are no clear guidelines to distinguish the cases in which physicians should make their own determinations from the cases in which they should not.

Whether a judicial determination of incompetency is necessary is part of the larger issue of whether resort should be had to the courts at a number of possible points in the medical decisionmaking process. (The merits and disadvantages of judicial involvement are discussed in Section 5.4.)

5.4 Procedural Issues

Choosing a Surrogate

Once a patient is determined to be incompetent, whether the determination is made clinically or judicially, someone must be selected to make decisions for the patient. This person is referred to generically as a surrogate (31). Particular kinds of surrogates include a guardian, who is a court-appointed surrogate, and a proxy, who is a surrogate selected by the patient himself. The phrases legal representative or legally authorized representative are sometimes used in the same general way as the term surrogate (32). Occasionally, the terms committee or conservator are used to indicate a court-appointed surrogate. To further confuse the matter, occasionally the term surrogate denotes someone who is court-appointed. It is no wonder that there is so much uncertainty about a matter as important as how the surrogate is to be chosen when there is so much inconsistency over matters as simple as terminology.

When a court makes the determination of incompetency and appoints a guardian, it may ask health care personnel to recommend a guardian if no likely person—such as a close and concerned family member—is immediately in evidence. When the determination is made in the clinical setting, the selection of the surrogate falls to clinical personnel. It is doubtful that most health care institutions actually have formal procedures governing such matters. Issues such as whether it is the responsibility of the attending physician or of other hospital personnel, such as nursing or social service, to select a surrogate are decided on an ad hoc basis, probably without anyone giving much formal recognition to the process. One family member may have been more dominant than others in caring for the patient, dealing with personnel, and expressing concern. This person may have been making decisions for the patient before hospitalization or care were needed and naturally continues to do so when the need for more formal decision making arises.

In some states, statutes specify that particular family members are empowered to consent on behalf of incompetent patients (e.g., 33, 34; see generally 35). In such a case there is ordinarily no need for court appointment of a guardian, unless there is serious conflict among family members of equal degree of relationship. Presumably it is the responsibility of the attending physician, with guidance from the hospital administration, to determine which particular person qualifies under the statutory requirements in given cases.

There is one other way in which a surrogate may be selected, and that is by the patient before becoming incompetent. Through the use of legal instruments such as a durable power of attorney, or pursuant to a small but increasing number of statutes designed for this purpose, or by more informal means, patients may designate another to make medical decisions should they become incompetent (27, pp. 145–147; 36–38). These are referred to as advance directives—specifically, proxy directives, because through them patients appoint proxies. (Another kind of advance directive, an instruction directive, is discussed below.) The legitimacy of such designations is open to some question, except where they are made pursuant to statutes specifically enacted for the purpose. There are only a small number of cases that explicitly (39,40) or implicitly approve such practices, but a trend appears to be developing toward approval (41–43).

Two forces are pushing health care institutions to adopt more formal policies for surrogate selection and incompetency determination (44). The first stems from demographic trends. There are increasing numbers of elderly persons who though not incompetent simply because of age are more likely in fact to be incompetent due to chronic illness and to require a series of decisions to be made on their behalf over an extended period of time. The second force is legal. Increasing attention is being paid by courts, legislatures, regulators, and possibly prosecutors to procedures and standards for decision making, especially as regards life-sustaining treatment.

A more formal policy needs to address the question of who within the institutional structure should have the responsibility for formally designating a surrogate. Another necessity is to address the problem of how that person should make the designation. Although no precise formula can be established, guidelines can be created that focus on factors such as the absence or presence of a family relationship, the closeness of that relationship in law, and the closeness of that relationship in fact. Attention must also be given to situations in which patients either have no family or there are no available or concerned family members. It needs to be decided whether a friend, if one exists, may serve as a surrogate or whether in such a case judicial guidance will be sought.

For those situations in which there is no readily available person, either family or friend, guidelines should be established for whether the patient's physician or a nurse, social worker, or hospital administrator should, or even may, serve as a surrogate. At this time there is no law either explicitly permitting or preventing such a practice, though the possibilities for a conflict of interest are obvious. Nonetheless, in such cases there is often no one else who can or will serve as a surrogate. Governmental and nonprofit health and welfare agencies, which often are other likely candidates for providing surrogates, rarely have the resources or inclination to do so. Bank trust departments, the traditional source of guardians of an incompetent person's estate, are similarly reluctant and ill-equipped to become involved in making medical decisions.

How Should the Surrogate Decide?

Once a surrogate has been selected, by whatever means, the decisionmaking process should proceed much as it would if the patient were competent, with the surrogate participating in place of the patient. The ideal remains that embodied in the idea of informed consent: collaborative decision making, in this case between surrogate and physician.

The role of the physician is to provide the surrogate with information about the medical options, their risks, and their benefits. The ideal role of the surrogate is to interject the patient's values into the decisionmaking process, to the extent that they are known or knowable. Thus, an added responsibility of the surrogate, especially one who does not know the patient very well or at all, is to attempt to learn more about the patient. In the case of a patient who is incompetent but not uncommunicative, the surrogate may carry on conversations with the patient to the best of his or her ability, talk with others—friends and family— who knew or know the patient well, and otherwise attempt to learn about the patient's values, goals, hopes, and fears in general, and in particular with reference to the patient's medical condition, its prognosis, and the available treatments.

Thus, the decisionmaking process for incompetent patients ought to look very much as it should when the patient is competent, with the obvious exception that the surrogate plays the patient's role. But that is only a part of the issue. There is still the problem of substantive standards for decision making.

When competent patients make decisions for themselves, by definition they do so in accordance with their own sense of what is best for them. This is not to say that others will agree that the decision is best, or even good. Nor is it to say that if faced with the same decision at a different time, the patient would necessarily make the same decision, or that if there were a succession of decisions there would necessarily be a logical consistency among them. People's goals, values, preferences, and desires are not so certain, consistent, and known even to themselves that rationality of this kind will often be achieved.

Most commentators contend that the goal of decision making by surrogates should be to replicate the decision that patients would make for themselves if they were competent to do so (31, pp. 177–181; 45, p. 209). This ideal is far more easily stated than achieved, if only because many people cannot even say with much precision how they themselves would act in the future should a certain set of circumstances arise, let alone how someone else would. Nonetheless, people can and do leave evidence of their wishes so that others may attempt to carry them out, at least in a general sort of way.

Decision making by a surrogate on behalf of an incompetent patient that attempts to replicate the patient's own decision, guided by the patient's own values, goals, preferences, and wishes, is called substituted judgment (31, pp. 178–179). The substituted judgment standard can be implemented in several ways. The simplest and most unequivocal is for patients, while competent, to leave written instructions about the kind of care they would wish to have in the event that they become incompetent. This is known as an advance directive, specifically an instruction directive.

While useful, instruction directives have limitations. The more general they are, the less useful they may be. On the other hand, if they are too specific, they may not contemplate the particular decision with which the surrogate is faced.The value of an instruction directive can be enhanced if combined with a proxy directive— that is, the naming of a particular person to act as surrogate. If the proxy both knows the patient and has the benefit of the instruction directive, the patient's wishes may be more closely approximated than with an instruction directive alone.

If made in writing, an instruction directive may take several forms. It may be cast in the form of a durable power of attorney. The precise legal status of such a document remains uncertain, because statutes authorizing durable powers of attorney were not enacted with medical decision making in mind. No appellate court as yet has specifically approved their use for this purpose. A few states have specific statutes authorizing such use, and where they exist they should be utilized. If a patient is terminally ill and wishes to give instructions about care in the event of incompetency—the situation in which advance directives are most likely to be used— the majority of states have natural death acts, which permit directives to be given (46). However, many of these acts are hedged with qualifications that substantially limit their usefulness (47).

Instruction directives need not be made in writing. In fact, the status of oral directives is, ironically, more certain than that of written directives. A number of courts have enforced oral instructions from patients who have stated, while competent, that they would not wish to have certain kinds of life-sustaining treatment administered should they become incompetent and incurably ill (41, 42, 48–51). It is only because of that certainty that we can infer that a written one also is valid and enforceable.

The substituted judgment approach is a subjective one; its aim is to implement the subjective preferences of the patient about and for whom decisions must be made. As such, it is most consonant with the goals of the informed consent doctrine itself. However, in many cases—indeed, probably most—patients have not given either written or oral instructions. In these situations surrogates cannot be guided by the the patient's express wishes. Some other standard must be applied.

The traditional best interests standard—deciding according to the surrogate's views of what would benefit the patient most— common in medical decision making and in law too, was until quite recently the sole standard by which decisions were made on behalf of incompetent patients. Only in the last quarter-century or so— roughly the same period in which the informed consent doctrine was born and matured—has the best interests standard increasingly received competition from the substituted judgment approach. This is not surprising, since the same forces that have served as an impetus to the idea of informed consent have acted similarly in regard to decision making for incompetent patients, who presumably would wish to have decisions made for them in accordance with their values rather than someone else's.

The conflict between these two standards may be greater in theory than in practice. All surrogate decision makers are, in a general way, under a duty to act in the best interests of incompetent patients. The difficulty with the best interests standard is not in the statement of it but in giving content to it. The substituted judgment approach is, in fact, one way of doing so. That is, a surrogate who makes a decision for an incompetent patient on the basis of that patient's instructions—written or oral, express or implied—is seeking to implement the patient's best interests *as that patient would have defined them*. Thus, the substituted judgment approach is merely one way in which the best interests standard is given content.

In the absence of such subjective advance directives from patients, content must be given to the best interests standard through the application of objective standards. Even if patients do not leave express directions about their health care, the patterns of their lives provide some, possibly substantial, information about their values, goals, preferences, and wishes that may prove useful to a surrogate. A decision based on such information can be called a limited-objective approach (44). Because there is often no bright line between one's express directives—especially when cast in a general way—and one's religious beliefs, ethical values, or lifestyle, the substituted judgment and the limited-objective best interests approaches shade into each other.

The limited-objective approach in turn stands in contrast to a pure-objective approach to determining best interests, which is used when the surrogate has no information whatsoever available about the patient that can serve as a guide, or when there is substantial reason to doubt the competency of the patient's previous choices. In these kinds of cases surrogates must make determinations based entirely on objective criteria—that is, they must make decisions that reasonable people would want made for them (44).

The Role of the Courts

There are a number of points in the process of decision making for incompetent patients when consideration might be given to seeking judicial guidance. Among the reasons for doing so are the fear of civil or criminal liability for an action taken without judicial sanction, a desire to protect patient autonomy, and a genuine desire for help in making the right decision.

The first point at which the courts might be consulted is in the determination of incompetency. If there is no serious question about a patient's competency, it may not be necessary to go to court, depending upon the precise statutory requirements and case law of the particular jurisdiction. In any event, customary practice is not to seek an adjudication of incompetency when a patient is clearly incompetent—for example, comatose.

The second point where judicial guidance may be sought is at the appointment of a surrogate. If an adjudication of incompetency has been sought and obtained, the surrogate will be appointed by the court. If incompetency is determined in the clinical setting, a surrogate will ordinarily be selected in that setting. Only when special circumstances arise—such as substantial and intractable conflict among potential candidates for the position of surrogate, or if there is no one at all to serve as surrogate—will judicial guidance be sought for the appointment of a surrogate, if it was not previously sought for the determination of incompetency.

Even if there has been no resort to the judicial process either for a determination of incompetency or the appointment of a surrogate, the existence of an advance directive from the incompetent patient may create a need for judicial guidance. Questions about the formal validity of the directive (e.g., whether a written document is a forgery) or its substantive validity (e.g., whether it requests an act that is illegal) may prompt the seeking of judicial review. Directives that are vague, confusing, internally conflicting, in conflict with the wishes of the surrogate, or in conflict with the current expressed wishes of the patient—incompetent though he or she may be—may also create a need for judicial review.

Assuming that none of the foregoing events have prompted recourse to the courts, a hearing may still be sought to review the substance of the decision made by the surrogate, especially if that decision is in serious conflict with what the attending physician or other professional staff believe to be medically or ethically appropriate. Even if there is no such disagreement, there may still be a legal requirement for judicial review, or if not a requirement, at least some concern whether the chosen course of action is legally sound.

The question of when there must be resort to the judicial process in medical decision making for incompetent patients has been infrequently addressed by the courts. The issue rarely arises, largely because the medical profession has unspoken and unwritten customs governing decision making for incompetent patients that ordinarily operate smoothly. Only when some difficulty with customary practice occurs is guidance from courts sought.

Although in theory there are a number of discrete points at which judicial review might be sought, in practice they tend to overlap or collapse into a single question. The questions of adjudication of incompetency and selection of a surrogate, though conceptually distinct, are usually resolved as a single issue. From the perspective of the participants in the decisionmaking process, there is often a single question to be addressed, to which all other questions are subordinate: What treatment, if any, should be provided? If this overriding question can be resolved without intractable conflict among the interested parties (family, patient, friends, attending physician, house staff, nurses, social workers, technicians, administrators—some or all of whom may have a say in a particular case) the issue of judicial review is unlikely to arise. Such recourse is only sought when some hitch develops—for example, a patient who is not clearly incompetent and is refusing medically indicated treatment (9, 52–54); conflict between the family's and the patient's wishes (52); conflict among family members about the proper course of treatment (31); concern that the patient's surrogate is not acting in the patient's best interests (55–57); fear of civil or criminal liability (40, 44, 58); a conflict between the surrogate's decision and the ethical precepts of the attending physician (59); confusion over what a patient's substituted judgment would be (60).

Such problems are most likely to occur, it seems, in cases involving decisions about life-sustaining treatment and about involuntarily hospitalized psychiatric patients. In these areas a number of pitched battles have been fought since the late 1970s. The debates continue, though resolution seems to be slowly coming. The New Jersey Supreme Court has explicitly required that incompetency be determined judicially in cases involving the foregoing of life-sustaining treatment (43). In the context both of life-sustaining treatment and psychiatric treatment, the Massachusetts Supreme Court has required that the decisions of surrogates— either consenting to or refusing treatment—be subjected to judicial review (13, 61, 62). At the same time, in cases involving life-sustaining treatment, that court has also transformed what had originally seemed to be an ironclad rule of judicial review into a more flexible one, in so doing creating uncertainty about precisely when review is required (63). Massachusetts courts have also categorically exempted from judicial review decisions about writing DNR (do not resuscitate) orders (64, 65) on the ground that such decisions "present a question peculiarly within the competence of the medical profession," because in the case of terminally ill patients, "attempts to apply resuscitation, if successful, will do nothing to cure or relieve the illnesses which will have brought the patient to the threshold of death" (64). By and large, the few courts that have made any mention of the issue of judicial participation seem to take the position of being available for judicial review, but not requiring it (15, 39, 41, 43, 66–68).

The Advantages and Disadvantages of Judicial Review

The question of when judicial guidance should be sought has been the source of a great deal of debate in the courts and especially in the medical and legal literatures. Much of the controversy stems from the fact that to have judicial guidance, oversight, or review— whatever name is used—of medical decision making is substantially at odds with long-standing professional custom. Consequently, such guidance has the potential to cause a great deal of resentment and discomfort among physicians who believe that their prerogatives are being eroded or eliminated. In fact, in many respects judicial review of medical decision making for incompetents often engenders adverse reactions from the medical profession similar to its reactions to the requirement to obtain informed consent from competent patients. Both informed consent and judicial review represent threats to physicians' freedom in making decisions about what kinds of treatment patients will receive. To the extent that both represent an interjection into the decision-making process of values that not only belong to persons other than the attending physician but also are nonmedical, they are perceived as undermining the authority of individual physicians and of the medical profession itself.

In addition, judicial participation in the process moves the locus of decision making out of a forum where physicians not only may control the process, but also can shield it from any substantial scrutiny by others. In fact, decision making within the clinical setting is all but invisible, whereas a judicial forum often exposes the process not merely to sunlight but to klieg lights. Not only is the content of the decisionmaking process now open to review, but the very fact that such decisions are made at all now becomes obvious, sometimes painfully so.

Although attempting to avoid legal liability is one of the motivations for seeking judicial review, it will not absolutely confer immunity (43, 63). In fact, absolute immunity will never be conferred on physicians or other health-care personnel when they are making a decision that involves the exercise of professional judgment. A judicial determination of incompetency will assure that a physician may rely upon the decisions of a judicially appointed guardian without incurring liability for battery for unauthorized treatment, as long as the guardian has consented. This does not constitute an absolute grant of immunity from liability, because physicians will still be liable, criminally or civilly, to the same extent they would have been had they dealt directly with a competent patient. That is, if the physician fails to use reasonable care in making a diagnosis and thus recommends improper treatment, or fails to use reasonable care in providing treatment, there can still be liability for negligence if the patient is harmed as a result of the physician's conduct, regardless of the fact that the guardian may have consented to the conduct.

Similarly, physicians who disclose inadequate information to surrogates may be liable for failing to obtain informed consent. If they fail altogether to obtain consent from surrogates, they may be liable for battery for the unauthorized rendition of medical care. Finally, any conduct that would be criminal even if performed by a physician with the consent of the patient will likewise be criminal if performed with the consent of the surrogate; any criminal omission to treat will similarly be grounds for liability even if the surrogate consents to it.

Apart from questions of liability, there are other arguments for seeking or avoiding judicial review of surrogates' decisions. First, the logistics of obtaining judicial review argue against it. If a situation is not labelled an emergency, the matter is likely to be considered by the courts as a routine matter, which means that some delay, perhaps a great deal, may occur. Delay may not threaten a patient's life or health, but it may impose physical pain, emotional suffering, and added cost, and contribute to the demoralization of professionals, patients, and families. (If the situation is an emergency, a determination of incompetency is not needed since the emergency exception will authorize the physician to provide necessary treatment at least to maintain the status quo.)

Resort to the courts can also incur financial costs, sometimes substantial, for both the hospital and the patient or family. In some jurisdictions legal counsel for both parties will be mandatory, and where it is not mandatory it will usually be desirable. If the issue is serious enough to require judicial attention, it would be unwise to enter judicial proceedings unrepresented by an attorney. Furthermore, even if judicial review is relatively simple to obtain in a particular case, the judicial system is probably not well equipped to handle the large number of cases that would arise if all such cases were subjected to judicial review.

Beyond these logistical matters is the question of whether courts are well suited to decision making of this kind. A good theoretical argument can be made that the business of courts is to make decisions, but in practice judges often feel uneasy and insecure about their own ability to make what they view as medical decisions (30). The result is substantial deference to professional medical judgment. If courts merely rubber-stamp professional decisions, much of the value of the judicial forum is lost (69).

However, some value does remain. What appears in the vast majority of cases to be rubber-stamping of professional decisions may be an acknowledgment that the time-honored method of decision making involving physician and family usually does result in decisions that are in an incompetent patient's best interests. But usually does not mean always. The courts exist to identify those cases in which professional judgment or family inclinations have gone astray, which can only be accomplished by the review of all cases. It may be, however, that the costs imposed by review of all cases in order to identify a few incorrectly decided ones is too high a price to pay. There may be other ways of identifying such cases at a lower cost.

Ethics Committees

The inadequacies of the existing method of making decisions for incompetent patients have long been apparent. The primary deficiency is that the process is riddled with uncertainty about two issues. First, what substantive decisions are legally and ethically acceptable? Second, assuming that a decision is a legitimate one, what are the appropriate procedures for making it? Physicians, and the hospital or nursing home administrators to whom they usually turn for advice in such matters, are unclear about when they are entitled, without fear of legal liability and without violating professional ethics, to rely on decisions to terminate care made by competent patients, or family members of incompetent patients. Physicians' concerns are embodied in the simple question they often ask: Do we have to go to court?

Only the attorneys to whom hospital administrators sometimes turn for advice seem to have a certain answer, but theirs is an answer born more of fear than of knowledge of the law. Their advice, in essence, is that when in doubt, it is best to play it safe and go to court or continue to provide treatment even if patients or their families object.

Judicial resolution of these kinds of questions rarely occurred prior to recent times, and such recourse has not always been well received by the courts. In 1966, a New York trial court judge, presented with the question of whether the gangrenous limb of an 80-year old woman should be amputated at the request of her lawyer son, over the objection of her physician son, opined against

> the current practice of members of the medical profession and their associated hospitals of shifting the burden of their responsibilities to the courts, to determine, in effect, whether doctors should proceed with certain medical procedures [and the] ultra-legalistic maze we have created to the extent that society and the individual have become enmeshed and paralyzed by its unrealistic entanglements (30)!

Although somewhat intemperate, the judge's remarks are not hard to understand when viewed as a symptom of his frustration, born of uncertainty as to what the law really is. It is not only physicians, hospital administrators, and their lawyers who are uncertain about how decisions should be made and what decisions are acceptable. Indeed, they are in the dark as much as they are largely *because* of the absence of legislative guidance or authoritative judicial precedents.

The exasperation expressed by the New York judge was not repeated in recorded legal annals for another decade, until the *Quinlan* case in 1976. Again, a court was confronted with the problem of how decisions should be made for incompetent patients. In more measured tones, the New Jersey Supreme Court recommended that a hospital ethics committee review such decision making rather than requiring judicial review:

> We consider that a practice of applying to a court to confirm such decisions would generally be inappropriate, not only because that would be a gratuitous encroachment upon the medical profession's field of competence, but because it would be impossibly cumbersome (58).

The court based its recommendation for the use of an ethics committee on a law review article (70). The court obviously believed that such committees existed; in fact they did not. Furthermore, the term ethics committee was somewhat of a misnomer in light of the function that the court assigned to it—namely, confirmation of the patient's prognosis.

Nonetheless, the idea of using ethics committees instead of courts to make such decisions captured the imagination of many physicians and hospital administrators, who saw it as a way of avoiding unwanted inconvenience, expense, and perhaps publicity, and who often resented "the law" telling them how to practice medicine. The suggestion, however, was not as welcome in judicial circles. The Massachusetts Supreme Court expressed outright disdain for the use of ethics committees in lieu of judicial review, but did acknowledge the potential usefulness of such a committee as an adjunct to judicial decision making:

[T]he [trial] court judge may, at any step in these proceedings, avail himself or herself of the additional advice or knowledge of any person or group. . . . We believe it desirable for a judge to consider [the views of an ethics committee] wherever available and useful to the court. We do not believe, however, that this option should be transformed by us into a required procedure. We take a dim view of any attempt to shift the ultimate decisionmaking responsibility away from the duly established courts of proper jurisdiction to any committee, panel or group, ad hoc or permanent. Thus, we reject the approach adopted by . . . *Quinlan* . . . (13).

Even the New Jersey Supreme Court, which first catapulted the idea of ethics committees into the public arena, seems to have backed off from its initial enthusiasm. In the *Conroy* case, decided almost a decade after *Quinlan,* the court decided not to rely upon ethics committees to make or review decisions about withdrawing life-sustaining treatment from patients in nursing homes, on the ground that "[f]ew nursing homes . . . have 'ethics' or 'prognosis' committees" (43). The same was true—even more so—of hospitals a decade earlier, and did not deter the same court from pronouncing their utility then.

The discussion about establishing and using ethics committees for decisionmaking purposes continues to grow. It is largely positive, though there are occasional notes of caution and outright opposition. Ethics committees have been proposed for use in cases not only of incompetent, terminally ill patients but also competent terminally ill, and incompetent, nonterminally ill patients. Their use has been recommended to address questions about the determination of competency, the choice of a surrogate, and the appropriateness of honoring advance directives and current treatment decisions.

Besides operating within the confines of a particular health-care institution to review decisions about foregoing life-sustaining treatment, several other functions have been proposed for ethics committees. These functions may turn out to be just as important as the former. Indeed, because they are less controversial, they may, in the long run, become the primary functions of ethics committees.

In addition to, or possibly instead of, individual case consultation and review, ethics committees can play important roles in education and policy making. Education takes place at several levels.

The simplest is the self-education that committee members deliberately or necessarily undergo through committee service. Similarly, those who bring cases to committees for review—whether health-care professionals or patients and families—are also educated in the process. The committee may also make conscious efforts to provide more formal educational programs for itself, health-care professionals, patients and families, or possibly the community the hospital serves.

In their initial stages, ethics committees may deal with cases on an ad hoc basis. As their workload increases and their members become more sophisticated and knowledgeable, they will almost inevitably consider drafting policies for use in their health-care institution, in order to provide guidance for the resolution of future cases perhaps without resort to the committee for advice. Such policies also serve an educational function and help to provide some consistency in how decisions are made within the hospital or nursing home. In jurisdictions where there is no law to provide guidance about foregoing life-sustaining treatment, or where the law fails to address many important issues, institutional policies may play an important role in the development of professional standards that in the event of litigation may aid in the resolution of the dispute (45, p. 209).

Conclusion

Decision making for incompetent patients poses great problems for all concerned. Physicians may be stymied by such issues as the standards and procedures to use in determining whether or not a patient is incompetent, who should make decisions for incompetent patients, and when to honor or override surrogate decisions. The fear of legal liability may subtly pervade the atmosphere in which such questions arise, probably inclining physicians to err on what they believe to be the safe side by providing treatment when in doubt. In fact, the prospect of liability is extremely remote. Moreover, liability may be as much a risk of providing unwanted treatment as of not providing medically indicated treatment. Finally, decision making for incompetent patients may be complicated by conflicts among professional staff, family members and friends of the patient, and members of these two groups.

Despite the large number of pitfalls that do exist, reported judicial cases involving treatment of incompetent patients are relatively few compared with the large number of physician-patient contacts. When such cases do arise, more often than not they involve decisions to forego life-sustaining treatment. Such cases may be even more emotionally charged and the fear of legal liability runs even higher. It is not likely that a consensus will soon be reached over what procedures to follow and what substantive standards to apply. In the meantime, the present uncertainty demands special sensitivity and diplomacy on the part of physicians and other health-care personnel in dealing with dying patients and their families.

References

1. Pratt v. Davis, 118 Ill. App. 161, 168, 174–75 (1905), *aff'd* 79 N.E. 562 (Ill. 1906).

2. Schloendorff v. Society of New York Hospital, 105 N.E. 92 (N.Y. 1914).

3. In re Long Island Jewish-Hillside Medical Center, 342 N.Y.S.2d 356, 358 (Sup. Ct. 1973).

4. Wilkins LP: Children's rights: removing the parental consent barrier to medical treatment of minors. *Arizona State Law Journal* 1975:31–92.

5. Pilpel HF: Minors' rights to medical care. *Albany Law Review* 36:462–487, 1972.

6. Wadlington W: Minors and health care: the age of consent. *Osgoode Hall Law Journal* 11:115–125, 1973.

7. Roth LH, Meisel A, Lidz CW: Tests of competency to consent to treatment. *Am J Psychiatry* 134:279–284, 1977.

8. Appelbaum PS, Roth LH: Competency to consent to research: a psychiatric overview. *Arch Gen Psychiatry* 39:951–958, 1982.

9. E.g., In re Quackenbush, 383 A.2d 785, 788 (N.J. Super. 1978).

10. E.g., In re B., 383 A.2d 760, 762 (N.J. Super, 1977). But see Lane v. Candura, 376 N.E.2d 1232 (Mass. App. Ct. 1978).

11. Relf v. Weinberger, 372 F. Supp. 1196 (D.D.C. 1974).

12. Strunk v. Strunk, 445 S.W.2d 145 (Ky. 1969).

13. Superintendent of Belchertown State School v. Saikewicz, 370 N.E.2d 417 (Mass. 1977).

14. In re Weberlist, 360 N.Y.S.2d 783 (Sup. Ct. 1974).

15. Matter of Storar, 420 N.E.2d 64 (N.Y. 1981).

16. Moore v. Webb, 345 S.W.2d 239 (Mo. App. 1961).

17. Demers v. Gerety, 515 P.2d 645 (N.M. Ct. App. 1973).

18. Gravis v. Physicians & Surgeons Hosp., 427 S.W.2d 310 (Tex. 1968).

19. Grannum v. Berard, 422 P.2d 812 (Wash. 1967).

20. Sullivan MT: The dying person—his plight and his right. *New England Law Review* 8:197–216, 1972.

21. E.g., In re W.S., 377 A.2d 969, 972 (N.J. Super. 1977).

22. Drane JF: The many faces of competency. *Hastings Center Report* 15(2):17–21, 1985.

23. Roth LH, Appelbaum PS, Sallee R, et al.: The dilemma of denial in the assessment of competency to consent to treatment. *Am J Psychiatry* 139:910–913, 1982.

24. 42 U.S.C. §§ 405(j), 1383(a)(2).

25. Robertson JR: *The Rights of the Critically Ill.* New York, Bantam, 1983.

26. Baron CH: Assuring "detached but passionate investigation and decision": the role of guardians ad litem in Saikewicz-type cases. *American Journal of Law & Medicine* 4:111–130, 1978.

27. President's Commission for the Study of Ethical Problems in Medicine and Biomedical and Behavioral Research: *Deciding to Forego Life-Sustaining Treatment: Ethical, Medical and Legal Issues in Treatment Decisions.* Washington, D.C., U.S. Government Printing Office, 1983.

28. Capron AM: Informed consent in catastrophic disease research and treatment. *University of Pennsylvania Law Review* 123:340–438, 1974.

29. Brakel SJ, Parry J, Weiner BA: *The Mentally Disabled and the Law.* Chicago, American Bar Foundation, 1985.

30. Matter of Nemser, 273 N.Y.S.2d 624 (Sup. Ct. 1966).

31. President's Commission for the Study of Ethical Problems in Medicine and Biomedical and Behavioral Research: *Making Health Care Decisions: The Ethical and Legal Implications of Informed Consent in the Patient-Practitioner Relationship.* Vol. 1, *Report.* Washington, D.C., U.S. Government Printing Office, 1982.

32. U.S. Department of Health & Human Services: Protection of Human Subjects. *45 Code of Federal Regulations Part 46.*

33. La. Rev. Stat. Ann. § 40:1299.53 (West 1977).

34. Utah Code Ann. § 78–14–5(4) (1977).

35. Meisel A, Kabnick LD: Informed consent to medical treatment: an analysis of recent legislation. *University of Pittsburgh Law Review* 41:407–564, 1980.

36. 20 Pa. Cons. Stat. Ann. § 5603(h) (Purdon Cum. Supp. 1985).

37. Cal. Civil Code § 2433 (West Cum. Supp. 1986).

38. Del. Code Ann. tit. 16 § 2501 et seq. (1983).

39. John F. Kennedy Memorial Hospital v. Bludworth, 452 So.2d 921 (Fla. 1984).

40. Saunders v. State, 492 N.Y.S.2d 510 (Sup. Ct. 1985).

41. Bartling v. Superior Court, 209 Cal. Rptr. 220 (Ct. App. 1984).

42. Matter of Eichner, 420 N.E.2d 64 (N.Y. 1981).

43. Matter of Conroy, 486 A.2d 1209 (N.J. 1985).

44. Meisel A, Grenvik A, Pinkus RL, Snyder JV: Hospital guidelines for deciding about life-sustaining treatment: Dealing with health limbo. *Crit Care Med* 14:239–246, 1986.

45. Veatch RM: *A Theory of Medical Ethics.* New York, Basic Books, 1981.

46. *The Physician and the Hopelessly Ill Patient: Legal, Medical and Ethical Guidelines.* New York, Society for the Right to Die, 1985.

47. The California Natural Death Act: an empirical study of physicians' practices. *Stanford Law Review* 31:913–945, 1979.

48. Matter of Lydia E. Hall Hospital, 455 N.Y.S.2d 706 (Sup. Ct. 1982).

49. Severns v. Wilmington Medical Center, 421 A.2d 1334 (Del. 1980).

50. Leach v. Akron Medical Center, 426 N.E.2d 809 (Ohio Com. Pleas. 1980).

51. Tune v. Walter Read Army Medical Hosp., 602 F. Supp. 1452 (D.D.C. 1985).

52. Lane v. Candura, 376 N.E.2d 1232 (Mass. App. Ct. 1978).

53. State Department of Human Resources v. Northern, 563 S.W.2d 197 (Tenn. Ct. App. 1978).

54. Matter of Schiller, 372 A.2d. 360 (N.J. Super. 1977).

55. Custody of a Minor, 393 N.E.2d 836 (Mass. 1979).

56. Matter of Hoffbauer, 393 N.E.2d 1009 (N.Y. 1979).

57. In re Sampson, 317 N.Y.S.2d 641 (Family Ct. 1970).

58. Matter of Quinlan, 355 A.2d 647 (N.J. 1976).

59. Gutheil TG, Appelbaum PS: Substituted judgment and the physician's ethical dilemma: with special reference to the problem of the psychiatric patient. *J Clin Psychiatry* 41:303–305, 1980.

60. Gutheil TG, Appelbaum PS: The substituted judgment approach: its difficulties and paradoxes in the mental health setting. *Law, Medicine and Health Care* 13:61–64, 1985.

61. Matter of Roe, 421 N.E.2d (Mass. 1980).

62. Rogers v. Commissioner, 458 N.E.2d 308 (Mass. 1983).

63. Matter of Spring, 4905 N.E.2d 115 (Mass. 1980).

64. Matter of Dinnerstein, 380 N.E.2d 134 (Mass. App. Ct. 1983).

65. Custody of a Minor, 434 N.E.2d 601 (Mass. 1982).

66. Barber v. Superior Court, 195 Cal. Rptr. 484 (Ct. App. 1983).

67. Guardianship of Barry, 445 So. 2d 365 (Fla. Ct. App. 1984).

68. In re L.H.R., 321 S.E.2d 716 (Ga. 1984).

69. Pleak R, Appelbaum PS: The clinician's role in protecting patients' rights in guardianship proceedings. *Hosp Community Psychiatry* 36:77–79, 1985.

70. Teel K: The physician's dilemma; a doctor's view: what the law should be. *Baylor Law Review* 27:6–9, 1975.

6

Rules Governing Patients' Redress in the Courts

The legal requirements for clinicians to obtain informed consent reviewed in the preceding chapters represent one side of the law of informed consent. The evolution of the legal doctrine was driven by the demands of patients for redress for injuries, and a considerable amount of attention has been given by courts and legislatures to the questions of when and how compensation might be obtained. This chapter provides an overview of the law's approach to these issues.

In some important respects, the distinction between the law as it applies to the physician engaged in medical decision making with a patient and the law as it applies to that same patient who later seeks compensation in the courts is an artificial one. Insofar as the idea of informed consent is not embraced voluntarily by the medical profession, but is adhered to in large part to avoid the likely consequences of failure to observe the legal rules, physician behavior will be shaped not only by the rules themselves but also by the way they are enforced.

If, for example, the rules governing the means of redress were complex, time-consuming, and unlikely to yield the desired compensation, few injured patients would pursue a judicial remedy.

As a result, physicians would eventually realize that adverse consequences were unlikely to follow from a failure to observe the relevant rules and, except to the extent that they had accepted the ethical theory of informed consent, their adherence to the doctrine would crumble. Some critics of the present system contend that this has already happened.

On the other hand, rules that make recovery easier and more certain would be likely to encourage compliance with the requirements for informed consent. Differential emphasis by the courts on particular kinds of lapses by clinicians might also shape their actions accordingly.

Thus, the legal issues addressed in this chapter, although framed in legal terminology, must be seen as important (some would argue crucial) determinants of the ultimate impact of the legal theory of informed consent.

6.1 Theory of Recovery

The law of informed consent represents the application to medical practice and medical research of principles of the law of torts. The kinds of interests protected by tort law are varied, as are the particular legal theories behind that protection. So varied, in fact, are these interests that one legal scholar concluded that there is no such thing as a single law of torts, but only an unconnected set of pigeonholes into which the conduct of one who causes injury to another must be fit before the law will afford a remedy for that injury (1, p. 3). Among the interests tort law protects are the interests of the individual in freedom from harm to person, property, and reputation. In addition, tort law serves broad social goals such as the compensation of injured persons, the deterrence of harm-causing conduct, and the punishment of those who cause such conduct. In the last quarter-century, an increasingly prominent goal of tort law has been the efficient allocation of economic resources. This goal has been accomplished by requiring harm-causing activities to internalize previously externally borne accident costs that arise from the conduct of those activities.

Since the middle of the nineteenth century, tort law has accom-

plished these goals through two predominant theories of liability—
intentional tort and negligence. (A third theory, strict liability, has
gradually gained ascendance in some areas of conduct, including
some areas related to medical practice, but the informed consent
doctrine is traditionally associated with the first two theories.) As
their names suggest, these theories are designed to remedy injuries
intentionally or negligently caused respectively. Since physicians
intentionally cause harm to patients only rarely, the intentional
tort theory might seem inapropos. Nonetheless, this theory is
where the informed consent doctrine has its legal roots, because
of some subtleties attendant to the theory of intentional
torts.

Battery

There are a number of intentional tort theories—assault, battery,
and false imprisonment are the most common. But the one most
relevant to informed consent cases is battery. A battery occurs
when one person engages in conduct that is intended to, and does,
cause harmful physical contact with another person, as when, for
example, a person throws a punch in a barroom brawl or hits
someone with a rock. Less obviously, a battery is also committed
by contact, or *touching*, that is *offensive*, but not necessarily harmful—at least not in the sense of causing bodily injury (2,§18).
Contact with another person is ordinarily considered offensive if
it occurs without the consent of the person being touched. Thus,
a physician who fails to obtain a patient's consent to a medical
procedure that involves a touching of the patient commits the tort
of battery.

Perhaps because this reasoning is subtle, or perhaps because the
common meaning of the words used in this analysis differs from
their legal meaning, courts have long been uncomfortable with
imposing liability on physicians for intentional torts. Exceptions
occur when the facts of a particular case make it clear that the
physician intended to operate over a patient's express objection
or (less likely) actually intended harm to, and not merely offensive
nonconsensual contact with a patient. (In fact, it is apparent from
some judicial opinions that their writers were not even aware that
a battery can be accomplished when physicians intend to commit

offensive nonconsensual, but nonharmful, touchings as well as when they intend to bring about harmful contact.)

The early cases involving a lack of consent to treatment were generally dealt with under a battery theory. The same theory was generally applied in the precursor informed consent cases—that is, those cases in which the courts recognized that some legal wrong had been committed because of inaccurate or incomplete information from the physician to the patient, but in which their responses had not yet solidified into a universal and affirmative requirement of disclosure (see Chapter 3). In these cases the courts concluded that a battery took place if consent was based on a substantial misunderstanding, due to misinformation or a lack of information, of the nature of the procedure or its consequences to the patient (3).

Negligence

The other major theory of tort law relevant to informed consent is negligence. The law of negligence imposes very broad and general requirements upon most persons to act (or refrain from acting) in such a way that their behavior does not cause harm to other persons. In our various roles as pedestrians, vehicle operators, homeowners, business operators, employees, professionals, and others too numerous to mention, we are expected to comport ourselves in such a way as to avoid unintentional (as well as intentional) harm to others. Failure to use reasonable care in the conduct of such activities that results in harm to others constitutes negligence and requires the party causing the harm to compensate the victim for injuries to person, property, and—increasingly—emotions.

In order to recover under a negligence theory, the plaintiff must establish four *elements*: (1) that the defendant (injurer) had a duty to use reasonable care to prevent harm to the plaintiff; (2) that the defendant breached this duty; and (3) that the conduct that constituted the breach of duty was the cause of (4) harm (bodily injury, property damage, emotional harm, and/or economic loss) to the plaintiff.

Unintentional injuries to patients caused by physicians are remediable, if at all, as negligence. Such conduct is generally referred to as malpractice, but is more properly called professional negligence. A physician is under a duty to possess and exercise the care, skill, and training of what the law terms a reasonably prudent physician. If the physician fails in this duty and as a result a patient is injured, the physician has committed professional negligence. Examples range from performing the wrong type of surgery or leaving surgical implements in the patient's body to error in prescribing dosage or kind of medication or failure to take a thorough medical history leading to an incorrect diagnosis and delay in instituting treatment.

In all cases, the mere fact that the physician makes what retrospectively can be characterized as a mistake, or that the patient suffers bad results (or fails to obtain good results) from the physician's care is not the critical feature, though without it the patient has no right to obtain damages. What is critical is whether the physician's conduct measures up to legally acceptable standards. These standards are almost always determined by reference to the prevailing custom and practice in the medical profession.

In its origins, informed consent was treated as a kind of intentional tort rather than a form of professional negligence. Because the physician failed to give the patient adequate information about the potential consequences of the recommended procedure the patient's permission to proceed did not amount to consent. Thus, the physician's contact with the patient was offensive, because no consent was given, and if any harm to the patient resulted, damages could be recovered not only for the offense but, under well-accepted rules, for any harm that occurred as well.

Some of the early informed consent cases, however, were brought as professional negligence rather than battery cases. Unlike standard professional negligence cases in which the essence of a patient's complaint is that something the physician did (or failed to do) in the way of medical treatment caused harm, the basis of the complaint in an informed consent case is that the physician failed to provide the patient with adequate information. In an informed consent case, the physician's failure to use reasonable care consists not in the manner in which he performs the medical procedure, diagnoses illness, prescribes medication, or the like, but in making deficient disclosure to the patient.

Differences in Underlying Values

From the early 1960s to mid-1970s, a number of courts wrestled with the problem of whether an informed consent case ought to be treated as a battery or negligence. The difference between the two theories can be of substantial importance in terms of what a patient must prove, and whether or not damages are available at all. More fundamentally, the difference between the two theories reflects different underlying values that a legal doctrine of informed consent might seek to protect.

If lack of informed consent is remediable as a battery rather than negligence, a patient has a right to recover damages for inadequate disclosure alone, even if not physically injured by the physician's treatment. The wrong to the patient is the deprivation of a right of personal choice based upon adequate information, sometimes called a dignitary harm. In contrast, with negligence theory the right vindicated is the right to be free from bodily injury caused by substandard medical practice. If the negligence causes no bodily injury to the patient, no remediable wrong is considered to have occurred.

A further difference is that the focal inquiry under a battery theory is (at least nominally) whether or not consent was given. As stated above, in battery cases consent is not considered to have been given if the physician has failed to provide the patient with certain information (2, §892B[2]). In the earlier battery cases, the only information that the physician needed to provide to assure that the patient's assent amounted to consent was an explanation of the nature of the procedure (3). By the mid-1950s, however, courts could occasionally be found holding that it was necessary for the patient to be given a greater quantity of information in order for it to be said that consent had been given. Under a negligence theory, in contrast, the issue of consent takes a decidedly secondary role to the duty to disclose—measured by either a professional or lay standard. The inquiry concerning the adequacy of the disclosure is made central rather than being subsumed under the aegis of the term consent as it is used in the context of battery theory.

Such matters have implications for proof at trial. Under a negligence theory, patients must demonstrate what was adequate disclosure before they may attempt to show that there was inadequate disclosure, that the inadequate disclosure resulted in a decision to undergo treatment, and that the treatment caused physical injuries. They may need expert witnesses to establish some or all of these things. Under a battery theory recovery is far simpler, since all that need be demonstrated is that an invalid consent was obtained. For this expert witnesses need not be employed. Any ensuing harm will be deemed to be causally related to the battery; separate proof that provision of information would have altered the decision to undergo treatment is not required.

Finally, the choice of battery or negligence may affect whether a case gets to court and whether the physician's professional liability insurance coverage is available to reimburse injured patients. Statutes of limitation, which establish the interval within which a suit must be filed after a harm comes to light, differ for battery and negligence. These issues usually mean that a negligence theory is more favorable to plaintiffs. Furthermore, malpractice policies ordinarily do not provide coverage for intentional torts, so a patient suing under a battery theory would not have access to this potential pool of funds for compensation.

The dispute over whether a lawsuit alleging lack of informed consent ought to be treated as a battery or as professional negligence has slowly withered away. By the mid-1970s, almost all states that had considered the question had concluded that inadequate disclosure is actionable only as professional negligence, not battery. At the same time, the administration of therapy without any consent at all, or outside the scope of the consent given, is still actionable as a battery (4).

The predominance of negligence theory appears to have been based largely on judicial reluctance to stigmatize physicians with the label of having committed a battery, lumping them into the same category as barroom brawlers, rather than on any clear analysis of the differential impact of one option or the other.

Regardless of the legal theory used to bring a lawsuit for lack of informed consent, the fundamental legal duties imposed by the doctrine have the same general contours. A physician is still obligated to disclose information about treatment and to obtain the patient's consent. However, battery theory is generally viewed as more conducive to successful suits by patients and thus more supportive of patients' self-determination. In fact, some commentators believe that the legal requirements of informed consent would be more carefully observed had the battery approach been widely adopted. On the other hand, negligence theories are thought to restrict suits against physicians, thereby encouraging them to be more controlling when medical decisions need to be made, and presumably favoring the value of health. Thus, substantially different consequences flow from one theory or the other. These consequences go to the heart of the interests served by the informed consent doctrine, the burdens it imposes on physicians, and the protections it affords to patients.

6.2 Causation

A lawsuit based on any tort theory requires that the plaintiff must show both that he or she was injured and the defendant caused the injury. In cases involving intentional torts such as battery, the requirements for establishing causation are simple. Causation is rarely an issue, and few if any of the early simple consent cases even mention it. Under negligence theory, causation can be far more problematic.

In informed consent cases there are actually two issues of causation, although few courts explicitly acknowledge them. One has received wide attention—it concerns the link between the physician's failure to disclose and the patient's consent. The other causation question, rarely acknowledged, involves the link between the physician's provision of treatment and the patient's injury. We refer to the latter as injury-causation and the former as decision-causation.

Injury-Causation

When a patient is worse after treatment than before, it is not always clear whether the treatment was the cause of the worsened condition. It may be that the treatment was beneficial or neutral in effect, and the natural course of the illness or injury was responsible for the deterioration. Injury-causation requires the plaintiff to show that the medical procedure performed by the defendant led to the injury. This requirement is merely a specific instance of the general one in negligence cases that the plaintiff prove *cause-in-fact*—that is, that the defendant's conduct was the actual (as opposed to legal) cause of the plaintiff's injury. Ordinarily, this requires plaintiffs to show that they would not have been injured if the defendants had exercised reasonable care, for example, had a correct diagnosis been made, or had medication side effects been monitored closely enough that the medication could have been stopped before they became irreversible.

Sometimes an injury is produced by more than one causal agency. Where that is the case, it is often impossible for plaintiffs to demonstrate that they would not have been injured if a particular defendant had not been negligent. For example, suppose a plaintiff had been simultaneously shot and killed by two careless hunters who thought they were shooting at a deer. If either bullet alone would have killed the plaintiff, both hunters could go free despite their negligence, because the plaintiff would have been killed even if one of the hunters had not been negligent. Each hunter could argue that his or her act alone was not a necessary cause of the harm.

To avoid blatantly unjust situations of this sort, when more than one causal agent is involved, a plaintiff must demonstrate only that the defendant's failure to use reasonable care was a *substantial factor* in bringing about the injury. In professional negligence cases the same rule is applied. If a patient's injury is caused in part by the underlying illness or injury and in part by the medical intervention, cause-in-fact is established by the medical intervention being found to have been a substantial factor in producing the injury.

Courts and legislatures that have recognized the problem of injury-causation in informed consent cases have sometimes done so under the name of proximate cause—that is, a finding that the negligent act was sufficiently related to the injury to be a legal cause. This requirement, by whatever name, has been recognized explicitly in only a few jurisdictions, probably because it has been taken for granted as a necessary aspect of any action based on a negligence theory of liability (4).

Proof of injury-causation will generally require that the plaintiff produce expert testimony that it was the defendant's conduct, and not the plaintiff's original illness or injury, that caused the plaintiff's injury. For example, an expert might testify that chloramphenicol has been shown to cause aplastic anemia, and that the patient who received this drug did in fact die as a result of aplastic anemia, not the underlying infection. In some cases the common experience of laypersons may be adequate to determine the cause of the injury, and expert testimony is not needed. The negligent amputation of the wrong limb by a surgeon is a good example.

Decision-Causation

This type of causation refers to the nexus between the physician's failure to disclose and the decision made by the patient. When it can be said that if the physician had made proper disclosure, a decision would have been made to decline treatment, decision-causation exists. The question that has troubled courts and commentators is whether an objective or subjective test should be applied in determining the relationship between the physician's nondisclosure and the patient's consent to treatment. Under an objective test, the plaintiff must prove that the undisclosed information would have led a reasonable person to decline treatment; under a subjective test, the plaintiff must prove merely that he or she would have refused treatment. An example of a subjective test is the Alaska informed consent statute, which states that the "health care provider is liable for failure to obtain the informed consent of a patient if . . . but for that failure [to inform,] the claimant would not have consented to the proposed treatment or procedure" (5). A subjective test presents a lesser obstacle to recovery.

Prior to *Canterbury* v. *Spence,* courts had given very little attention to causation in informed consent cases (6). While courts considering the problem both before and after *Canterbury* agreed that causation exists only when disclosure of risks (or conceivably other information, such as alternatives) would have resulted in a decision to forego the treatment, the pre-*Canterbury* courts generally did not address the problem of whether causation is to be found by reference to an objective (reasonable person) or subjective (the particular patient) standard. Many commentators assumed that the subjective test should be applied (7–11). The courts concurred, though seemingly unaware of the issue (12).

Since the lead set in *Canterbury,* however, a subjective test has been rejected by most courts. The reason has been that a subjective analysis calls for the jury to credit the plaintiff's answer to a hypothetical question—for example, "Mr. Smith, if Dr. Jones had told you that you might lose motion in your arm as a result of this procedure, would you have gone through with it?" Such a question "places the physician in jeopardy of the patient's hindsight and bitterness"(6). On the other hand, the objective test has been criticized on the ground that it dilutes the patient's right of self-determination by honoring it only to the extent that the patient's judgment conforms to that of a reasonable person (13). The majority of courts and legislatures that have addressed the issue have adopted an objective test (14, pp. 206–245).

There is, however, a serious problem with this line of reasoning. Under an objective test, plaintiffs still may testify as to what they actually would have done had they been properly informed. Although such testimony will not definitively settle the decision-causation issue, the jury is entitled to consider the plaintiff's views. The *Canterbury* court, in rejecting a subjective test of causation, was skeptical of the plaintiff's ability to admit, after the fact, that he would have elected treatment even if adequate disclosure had been made. For the same reason that the *Canterbury* court was skeptical, it is reasonable to assume that most jurors will also be skeptical. Because it is the jury's function to evaluate all the evidence and to weigh the credibility of witnesses, there is ample opportunity for jurors to apply this natural skepticism. Thus, the fear of the courts may be overstated, if not misplaced.

Because the doctrine of informed consent is premised on the right of persons to make decisions about what medical care they wish to undergo, regardless of the soundness of their reasons, the subjective test of decision-causation is far more consonant with the underlying rationale for informed consent than the objective test. By conditioning the availability of compensation on the congruence between the patient's own decision and what a so-called reasonable person would have decided, the objective test undercuts a patient's right of self-determination. It is not difficult to understand why this test has been favored. As *Canterbury* indicates, and as other cases have agreed, it is unlikely that medical-accident victims would thwart their own chances to obtain compensation—no matter how much good faith we are willing to ascribe to them—by testifying that even had they been properly informed, they would still have consented.

To the best of our knowledge, no court has ever mentioned the possibility of applying any other type of test, nor have the legislatures. An attractive alternative is a material factor test, under which the jury would have only to find that the information withheld was material to the decision-making process. The use of a material factor test might pacify critics of both the objective and subjective tests. Patients would no longer be required to state that had disclosure been complete, they would have foregone treatment; the jury would no longer be required to evaluate the credibility of that statement. If the jury simply found that the undisclosed information would have been important, even if not determinative, it could find the necessary causal connection to have been proved.

The insistence on a demonstration of decision-causation stems from the unwillingness of the courts to view inadequate disclosure alone as a harm to a patient. This constitutes the strongest judicial resistance to recognizing that a patient can be wronged by a physician's behavior— specifically, inadequate disclosure—even when not physically harmed (13). This resistance conflicts with a fundamental purpose of the idea of informed consent: the protection and promotion of human dignity.

6.3 Procedural Aspects of Litigation

In a lawsuit based on a claim of lack of informed consent, the patient-plaintiff has the burden of producing evidence on each element of the *prima facie* case. There are four elements in all, as in any cause of action based on a negligence theory: duty, breach of duty, causation, and damages. (See Section 6.1.) To fulfill some of these elements, the plaintiff will need to produce the evidence of expert witnesses.

First, the patient needs to establish that the defendant-physician owed the patient a legal duty. This question is ordinarily one of law, decided by the court rather than the jury. Duty is not often at issue in informed consent cases. It has been established as a matter of law in all American jurisdictions that when a doctor-patient relationship exists, the physician owes the patient duties of disclosure and obtaining consent before treatment may be commenced.* Sometimes, however, there is a question about whether or not a doctor-patient relationship existed or whether it was the kind of doctor-patient relationship that required disclosure (17). This question can arise in a variety of ways. Often it occurs when one physician evaluates a patient and recommends a particular procedure, but refers the patient to another physician for its performance. A referring physician, as opposed to a treating physician, is not required to explain a procedure to a patient. Or sometimes this issue arises when a house officer inadequately informs a patient about a procedure but does not participate in its performance. In that case, it is again the treating physician who owes the patient a duty of reasonable disclosure (18).

Once duty is established—and usually there will be no dispute about this between the parties—the patient must introduce evidence of the second element of recovery, breach of duty. This element requires evidence about what the standard of care—that is, the standard of disclosure—is. In a jurisdiction that adheres to a professional standard of disclosure, the plaintiff must call an expert witness to establish what information a reasonably prudent physician would have disclosed (19,20). Where no other expert is available or willing to testify, the plaintiff may attempt to use the defendant-physician as his expert (21), but for obvious reasons this method is decidedly less effective. In order to complete the proof of breach of duty, the patient is also required to prove that the defendant did in fact fail to disclose information that a reasonably prudent physician would have disclosed.

In a jurisdiction adhering to a lay standard of disclosure, the plaintiff's proof is simpler: the plaintiff need only prove that information was not disclosed. The jury will decide on its own whether the information is of a type that would be material to the decision of a reasonable patient or (in some jurisdictions) the par-

---

*In Georgia, the required disclosure is limited to a description "in general terms [of] the treatment or course of treatment" (15). This requirement is so limited that it cannot properly be termed informed consent (16).

ticular plaintiff. In either case the plaintiff is likely to need an expert witness to establish that the undisclosed risk is actually associated with the particular treatment provided, or that a particular therapeutic option that was not discussed actually is an alternative to the treatment that was performed (12).

The patient must then prove the third element, causation. For injury-causation, the plaintiff-patient may again need the services of an expert witness (12). In addition, the trier-of-fact (usually a jury, but a judge if jury trial is waived) must be able to find decision-causation. In most jurisdictions where an objective standard of causation applies, this will mean that the trier-of-fact must find that reasonable persons would not have consented to treatment had they been told the very information that the physician neglected to disclose. For this aspect of the patient's case, no expert witness will be needed. In those few jurisdictions where a subjective standard applies, patients may introduce evidence that they themselves would not have consented to treatment had the omitted information in fact been provided. Evidence of this sort should also be admissible, though of less probative force, in a jurisdiction applying an objective test of causation (3).

Finally, the plaintiff must prove the fourth element: damages. In a case in which the omitted information concerned a risk of treatment, it must be this omitted risk that materialized and constituted the injury (22). If the physician neglected to inform the patient about an alternative treatment the plaintiff claims would have been chosen had it been explained, the plaintiff may recover for injuries even if informed of a risk that did materialize (23). The plaintiff may recover damages for any added medical expenses, any other out-of-pocket expenses occasioned by the injury, physical pain and mental suffering, and lost wages, salary, or income.

This evidence will satisfy the plaintiff's requirements as to the physician's duty of disclosure; however, the physician also has a duty to obtain the patient's consent, which the patient may also (or alternatively) claim has been breached. (If the claim is solely that the patient did not consent to treatment, rather than that inadequate information was provided, the cause of action should be for battery rather than negligence [24]). The fact that the patient may have signed a consent form is not necessarily conclusive evidence that legally valid consent was given (25–29). If the patient was unduly pressured into signing the form, the consent is not valid (2, §892B[3]). If the physician failed to use reasonable care in determining whether the patient understood the information, and in fact the patient did not, the patient has not given a legally valid consent (2, §892[B][2]). (See Chapter 9.)

No recovery may be obtained under an informed consent theory if the patient suffers no physical injury. Inadequate disclosure alone—that is the deprivation of the right of informed choice—is not a legally protected interest. In contrast, the failure to obtain consent, however well-informed the patient may be, does give rise to a cause of action under a battery theory for damages, even if the patient has not been physically harmed by the treatment, because the right of bodily integrity is a legally protected interest. Indeed, so well protected is the right not to be treated without consent that physicians have been held liable in battery for administering treatments that benefited patients but were not consented to (30–34).

It is the plaintiff's responsibility to introduce evidence on all of the above matters. If the plaintiff does so, a *prima facie* case has been established. If the plaintiff cannot produce enough information on these matters to meet this production burden, then the case will be dismissed, before the physician-defendant is required to introduce any evidence at all.

If the plaintiff does meet the production burden, the defendant-physician has two general choices. He or she may introduce no evidence and let the case go to the jury solely on the plaintiff's evidence. If the plaintiff's case is exceedingly weak, or if it is likely that information damaging to the physician will come out if the physician chooses to present evidence, the physician may prefer this alternative.

More likely, it will be to the physician's advantage to introduce evidence designed to weaken the plaintiff's case. This may be done in a number of ways, but there are two general approaches. The first is to introduce evidence that weakens one, several, or all of the elements of the plaintiff's *prima facie* case. The simplest way is to deny the plaintiff's claim that there was incomplete disclosure.

Testimony can be introduced—from the physician, for example, or a nurse, or the patient's spouse, if they were present when the doctor talked to the patient—that the patient was informed of the information the patient claims was not disclosed. Testimonial contests of this sort are a frequent occurrence in informed consent cases. Physicians are even permitted to testify about their usual disclosure practices for the type of information at issue (35,36). In a jurisdiction adhering to a professional standard of disclosure, the physician-defendant may introduce the evidence of expert witnesses as to what is customarily told patients about the procedure undergone by the patient. Similarly, on the issue of injury-causation, the defendant may introduce evidence tending to show that the patient's injury was not caused by the treatment. Decision-causation is more difficult to counter, unless the patient indicated in some way that he or she would have undergone the procedure in question regardless of the risks involved.

The second general approach is to establish an affirmative defense. Rather than merely attempting to weaken the plaintiff's evidence, this method admits, though only for argument's sake, that the defendant breached the duty of disclosure or the duty to obtain consent (or perhaps even both), but asserts that the physician was legally entitled to do so. In other words, the physician-defendant claims that one of the exceptions to obtaining informed consent applies: emergency, waiver, therapeutic privilege, or incompetency. (See Chapters 4 and 5.)

On each of these affirmative defenses, the physician bears the burden of making out a *prima facie* case. That is, the physician must introduce sufficient evidence for the trier-of-fact to find that the exception should apply (3, p. 104). If the physician fails to do so, these matters of defense cannot be considered by the jury.

References

1. Keeton WP, Dobbs DB, Keeton RE, Owen DG: *Prosser and Keeton on the Law of Torts.* 5th ed. St. Paul, West, 1984.

2. American Law Institute: *Restatement (Second) of the Law of Torts.* St. Paul, American Law Institute Publishers, 1965.

3. Meisel A: The expansion of liability for medical accidents: from negligence to strict liability by way of informed consent. *Nebraska Law Review* 56:51–152, 1977.

4. Meisel A, Kabnick LD: Informed consent to medical treatment: an analysis of recent legislation. *University of Pittsburgh Law Review* 41:407–564, 1980.

5. Alaska Stat. § 9.55.556(a) (Cum. Supp. 1983).

6. Canterbury v. Spence, 464 F.2d 772 (D.C. Cir. 1972).

7. Waltz JR, Scheuneman TW: Informed consent to therapy. *Northwestern University Law Review* 64:628–650, 1970.

8. Plant ML: An analysis of "informed consent." *Fordham Law Review* 36:639–706, 1968.

9. Informed consent in medical malpractice. *California Law Review* 55:1396–1418, 1967.

10. Informed consent as a theory of medical liability. *Wisconsin Law Review* 1970:879–898.

11. *Harvard Law Review* 75:1445–1449, 1962.

12. Shetter v. Rochelle, 409 P.2d 74 (Ariz. App. 1965).

13. Goldstein J: For Harold Lasswell: some reflections on human dignity, entrapment, informed consent, and the plea bargain. *Yale Law Journal* 84:683–703, 1975.

14. President's Commission for the Study of Ethical Problems in Medicine and Biomedical and Behavioral Research: *Making Health Care Decisions: The Ethical and Legal Implications of Informed Consent in the Patient-Practitioner Relationship.* Vol. 3, Appendices. Washington, D.C.: U.S. Government Printing Office, 1982.

15. Ga. Code Ann. § 31–9–6 (1985).

16. Young v. Yarn, 222 S.E.2d 113 (Ga. Ct. App. 1975).

17. Nicholson v. Curtis, 452 N.E.2d 883 (Ill. App. 1983).

18. Hill v. Seward, 470 N.Y.S.2d 971 (Sup. Ct. 1983).

19. Bly v. Rhoads, 222 S.E.2d 783 (Va. 1976).

20. German v. Nichopoulos, 577 S.W.2d 197 (Tenn. Ct. App. 1978).

21. Abbey v. Jackson, 483 A.2d 330 (D.C. Ct. App. 1984).

22. Cornfeldt v. Tongen, 262 N.W.2d 684 (Minn. 1977).

23. Logan v. Greenwich Hosp. Assoc., 465 A.2d 294 (Conn. 1983).

24. Cobbs v. Grant, 502 P.2d 1 (Cal. 1972).

25. Sard v. Hardy, 379 A.2d 1014 (Md. 1977).

26. Gassman v. United States, 589 F. Supp. 1534 (M.D. Fla. 1984).

27. Gordon v. Neviaser, 478 A.2d 292 (D.C. 1984).

28. Keane v. Sloan-Kettering Institute for Cancer Research, 464 N.Y.S.2d 548 (App. Div. 1983).

29. Siegel v. Mt. Sinai Hospital of Cleveland, 403 N.E.2d 202 (Ohio Ct. App. 1978).

30. Lloyd v. Kull, 329 F.2d 168 (7th Cir. 1964).

31. Bailey v. Belinfante, 218 S.E.2d 289 (Ga. App. 1974).

32. Mohr v. Williams, 104 N.W. 12 (Minn. 1905).

33. Rolater v. Strain, 137 P. 96 (Okla. 1913).

34. But see Buzzell v. Libi, 340 N.W.2d 36 (N.D. 1983).

35. In re Swine Flu Immunization Products Liability Litigation, 533 F. Supp. 567 (D. Colo. 1980).

36. Sauro v. Shea, 390 A.2d 259, 265 n.2 (Pa. Super. 1978).

7

Critical Approaches to the Law of Informed Consent

As the preceding chapters demonstrate, the law of informed consent has been shaped by two primary sets of values: individualistic values that support autonomous decision making, and widely held values supporting health. The balance struck between these interests has been influenced heavily by the structure of the legal process, particularly the law of negligence.

The result has been a doctrine and a set of practices that compromise all values and satisfy none in their entirety. In this context, the extent of the debate over informed consent among health care practitioners, legal experts, and ethicists should come as no surprise. As long as one relies on a single, consistent perspective, it is remarkably easy to find critical things to say about informed consent. Those who would elevate any single value above all others, and steadfastly resist compromise, can usually offer a powerful, even devastating, analysis of the current state of affairs.

Commentators who have analyzed the law and practice of informed consent have generally represented one of three points of view: a perspective concerned with promoting individual autonomy; an approach that emphasizes the value of health; and a perspective that sees as primary the value of encouraging discourse and interaction between caregivers and patients. In this chapter we look at all three and assess their validity from a perspective that recognizes that the doctrine that must accommodate a number of competing interests and values.

7.1 The Autonomy-Oriented Critique

The most trenchant criticism of the state of informed consent law today focuses on the discrepancies between the goals highlighted by the ethical theories of informed consent—primarily, the enhancement of individual autonomy in making medical decisions— and the practical effects of the current system. Theorists of this school, most notably Jay Katz, are troubled by the failure of the current law to protect autonomy as fully as it might, and by what they see as a consistent pattern of subordinating patient autonomy to the interests of the medical profession (1; 2, pp. 48–84).

Katz traces this problem to the very cases that provided the foundation for the modern notion of informed consent. He points to the wording of the sentence in which the term informed consent was born, in the court's opinion in *Salgo* v. *Leland Stanford Jr. University Board of Trustees:* "[I]n discussing the element of risk a certain amount of discretion must be employed consistent with the full disclosure of facts necessary to an informed consent" (3). "Only in dreams or fairy tales," says Katz, "can 'discretion' to withhold crucial information so easily and magically be reconciled with 'full disclosure' " (1, p. 138).

For Katz, the courts' continual deference to medical paternalism, exemplified by their willingness to accept "a certain amount of [medical] discretion" (3) has most served to restrict the impact of the law of informed consent. Katz sees the so-called discretion reserved to physicians in *Salgo* as the forerunner of courts' further obeisance to the medical profession, expressed in their preference for a professional standard of disclosure and their acceptance of therapeutic privilege as an exception to the requirement of disclosure. (Both the professional standard of disclosure and therapeutic privilege limit the amount of information patients are likely to obtain and force them into reliance on their doctors' opinions.) Even those courts that have adopted a patient-oriented standard for disclosure have, in Katz's view, compromised the gain to patients' autonomy by choosing an objective (what a reasonable patient would have found material) rather than a subjective (what the actual patient the would have found material) standard of the informational needs of the patient. The same could be said in the area of causation (whether a patient would have been deterred from treatment had the information been disclosed), where the courts have again, by and large, accepted an objective rather than subjective standard.

Katz's argument that the current law of informed consent is insufficient to compel physicians to share information with patients is supported by a number of empirical studies. Observational research has suggested that physicians in hospital settings rarely provide any substantial information to patients about diagnostic and treatment decisions, with the exception of decisions to employ surgical or other invasive procedures (4; 5, pp. 316, 317). Outpatients may receive somewhat more information, but this is often provided after the treatment decision is made and geared more toward facilitating compliance than encouraging participation in decision making (4). Surveys show consistently that patients desire to have more information than physicians routinely provide (6, 7).

Why are the courts, despite their rhetoric supporting patients' self-determination, so willing to contribute to the perpetuation of this state of affairs by continuing to bow to medical judgment? Largely, Katz believes, because they share the medical profession's low opinion of most patients' ability to understand the issues involved in medical treatment and to reach a reasonable decision. "Judges toyed briefly with the idea of patients' self-determination," he concludes, "and largely cast it aside" (1, p. 170).

As disturbing as Katz finds judicial deference to medical discretion, he is equally perturbed about the incorporation of informed consent into the law of negligence. Were the failure to obtain informed consent to lead to redress in an action for battery rather than negligence, Katz believes that plaintiffs would have a much easier time proving their cases, and the medical profession would be more punctilious in its observance of the consent requirements. (See Chapter 6.) In battery, plaintiffs would not be required to prove adverse effects of a failure to disclose in order to obtain a favorable verdict (although physical harms would certainly affect the size of any damages awarded). Nor would the law of battery necessarily require plaintiffs to demonstrate that their decisions about medical care would have been different had appropriate disclosure taken place. The failure to provide adequate information would have been viewed as the harm to the patient; that is, a *dignitary injury*, or insult to the personhood of the patient; this concept probably comes as close as any other to embodying Katz's view of the underlying rationale for informed consent.

Despite Katz's position as the most prominent theorist and critic of informed consent law, he has never formulated a comprehensive legal alternative to the current system. He would presumably favor addressing informed consent as a matter of battery law, and the adoption of subjective, patient-oriented standards. But he appears to recognize that this reorientation, which itself is unlikely to take place, would not necessarily improve matters all that much. Allowing patients to sue for dignitary harms, while theoretically appealing, might not significantly increase the number of legal cases filed. Such harms are likely to be compensated with only minimal damages, and few patients (not to mention attorneys) can be expected to pursue cases in which their time and effort will go largely unrewarded (1).

An even more important obstacle, in Katz's view, is the ineffectiveness of law in changing physician behavior. He admits that what he sees as physicians' long standing antipathy to sharing information with their patients is likely to be little affected by legal rules at all. An identification with the moral basis of informed consent, which can be attained only by a careful reeducation of the medical profession, may be the only effective means of promoting patient participation in decision making (2, pp. 228–229).

Particular attention has been given to Katz's autonomy-based critique of informed consent law because he has presented the most thorough analysis of the doctrine and its applications. Numerous other commentators, many of them probably influenced by him, have echoed and amplified his charges. Some have focused on individual elements of informed consent law, such as the acceptance by courts of the notion of therapeutic privilege. (See Section 4.3.) They have argued for the abolition of the privilege or for its limitation—for example, by excusing nondisclosure only of the information that itself is thought likely to cause the expected harm, but continuing to require otherwise complete disclosure (8,9).

Another favorite target of legal commentators is the professional standard of disclosure, seen by many as a major limitation on the right of patients to receive relevant information. Schneyer has offered probably the most interesting objection, namely that the differing amounts of remuneration various procedures offer create such substantial conflicts of interest for physicians in informing their patients about the desirability of one over another that physicians cannot be trusted to establish the standards of disclosure (10). Schneyer believes that physicians, particularly surgeons, cannot separate their pecuniary interests from their fiduciary obligations to patients and will consistently recommend, and shape their disclosures to insure that patients select, those procedures likely to yield the highest rates of compensation. Although perhaps viewed skeptically when first proposed, Schneyer's analysis is likely to be given more credence now that the economic aspects of physicians' behavior are coming under extensive scrutiny. Schneyer's critique takes on added significance in light of the high degree of specialization of physicians. When the available options include procedures not performed by the physician with whom the patient is currently dealing, there is an economic disincentive for the physician to discuss those options, perhaps even an incentive not to see them as options at all.

Several commentators have offered more sweeping proposals for restructuring the law, especially to allow recovery for the infliction of dignitary harms. One calls for "the legislature . . . [to] fashion sanctions other than damages for injury, such as fines, probation, loss of license or other administrative penalties, which could be imposed on a sliding scale, depending on the gravity of the offense [of failing to disclose appropriate information]" (11). Another author calls for a system of noninsurable tort-fines that would have the desired punitive and deterrent effect on physicians (12). The problem of encouraging patients to pursue these remedies in the absence of the prospect of substantial recovery of damages, however, has not yet been solved.

Riskin, whose concern "is based primarily on a commitment to human dignity as a value transcending even physical health," has offered two other suggestions (12). The first would, in essence, adopt a partial battery approach to informed consent cases by eliminating the current requirement for plaintiffs to prove the element of causation, that is, that their behavior would have been different had full disclosure been accomplished. Under this proposal, any undisclosed risk that materialized would warrant the assessment of damages. Alternatively, Riskin would reduce the standard of causation to require plaintiffs merely to show that they *might* not have consented had full, appropriate disclosure been made. Both suggestions would cut deeply against the negligence theory on which informed consent law has been based to date, and would approximate a system of strict liability for undisclosed risks that in fact occur (13).

The difficulties faced by commentators who would substantially reconstruct the informed consent system are well demonstrated by Simpson, who argued for a change in focus from mere disclosure to insuring that patients actually understand what they have been told. He would require courts "to consider whether the physician has taken reasonable measures to ensure that the patient *understands* the information disclosed" (8). After a lengthy discussion of the importance of comprehension, however, Simpson backs away from suggesting a system that would require it. Fearful that patients who cannot comprehend the nature and risks of treatment or choose to remain ignorant might thereby be deprived of medical care (a concern that appears to have motivated some of the courts that considered this issue as well), Simpson concludes merely with a detailed list of items physicians would be required to disclose. If this disclosure were made, and patients were encouraged to ask questions, he would presume comprehension.

Goldstein arrives at a similar solution from very different premises (14). In what might be termed an anti-Kantian mode of reasoning, he has argued that an emphasis on patients' comprehension would only serve to undercut their autonomy. If comprehension were to be the touchstone, he fears that uncomprehending patients would have their decisions made for them by others. Believing that even so-called irrational patients should have the right to determine their own medical care, Goldstein would focus entirely on the disclosure by the physician, shunning any assessment of comprehension (or even competency), and allowing for the pursuit of compensation for dignitary harms.

The autonomy-based critics of informed consent command a

wide following in legal and bioethical circles. The appeal of their arguments lies in their ability to identify substantial compromises of patient autonomy in current approaches to informed consent. They have had relatively little impact on the development of the law because they have consistently failed to deal effectively with their opponents' competing concerns—primarily, that too close an adherence to self-determination might encourage the harassment of physicians in the courts and lead patients to make decisions that would adversely affect their health. Katz comes closest to acknowledging the existence of these competing concerns but dismisses them as unsupported by empirical data. Most courts and legislatures, however, remain convinced that subjective standards and recovery for dignitary harms would encourage lawsuits and recoveries for plaintiffs in a manner that would be unfair to physicians. Moreover, they are generally willing to allow physicians some scope for paternalistic intervention, in the belief that patients sometimes require (and perhaps even desire) decisions to be made for, rather than with, them. Nevertheless, the autonomy-based critics have done a great deal to alert both the legal and medical professions to the danger that the idea of informed consent might be lost in the process of creating legal rules to enforce it.

7.2 The Health-Oriented Critique

Few commentators who address the issue of informed consent lack the belief that their approach, if adopted, will enhance the health of patients. We use the term health-oriented critique to refer to the position that favors a relaxation of the current disclosure and consent requirements imposed on physicians. Before exploring this position, however, it may be of interest to consider arguments based on health-related values that find favor with some critics who support even more disclosure and patient participation than is mandated by the present law of informed consent.

The Proponents of Informed Consent

Eleanor Swift Glass has suggested that therapeutic benefits would result from a rigorously defined requirement for informed consent

(11). Arguing for patient-oriented standards of disclosure, administrative mechanisms for imposing sanctions on doctors who fail to provide adequate disclosure, and limitations on the therapeutic privilege, she maintains that these changes would improve the overall quality of health care. Informed consent was unnecessary, she claims, when doctors knew their patients for long periods of time and could, in making decisions for them, accurately reflect the patients' own value systems. Modern, technologically oriented medicine interferes with the development of such relationships, proving too many incentives for physicians to neglect the human aspects of their patients. As a result, physicians make poor decisions on behalf of patients they barely know, leading to the improper choice of treatments and poor patient compliance. If physicians are compelled to discuss therapeutic options, risks, and benefits with patients, the result will be that additional relevant information will be elicited, personalized and joint decision making by doctor and patient will be encouraged, and a greater sense of teamwork and therefore compliance on the patient's part will ensue. Empirical data in this area are problematic, but there are reasons to believe that the provision of appropriate information and collaborative decision making will enhance compliance (15). A complementary argument in favor of tighter informed consent requirements focuses on the benefits of reduced patient anxiety as a result of more complete disclosure (4), a suggestion supported by findings in studies of surgical patients (16).

The most cogent statement of the belief that increased patient participation in medical decision making will improve patients' health comes from the report on informed consent of the President's Commission for the Study of Ethical Problems in Medicine and Biomedical and Behavioral Research (17, pp. 42–44). The commission emphasized that health, or well-being, must be defined broadly, and that the inability to make decisions congruent with one's values constitutes an impediment to the subjective, and probbly objective, attainment of a state of well-being. In the commission's approach, well-being is seen as influenced by a combination of physical and psychological factors. A narrow focus on objective indicia of physical health, often characteristic of the medical profession's traditional approach, ignores the broader aspects of persons' satisfaction with their state of existence.

The Opponents of Informed Consent

The ground of health-related values has been seized most fervently, often with the support of the courts, by the opponents of informed consent. Unlike other commentators on informed consent, they often employ empirical data to substantiate their arguments. The scientific background of most of these persons perhaps leads them to confer legitimacy primarily on positions that can be supported with actual data. Ironically, the data relating to informed consent are generally so poor that few reliable conclusions can be drawn from them (18). We will not review these data in detail, but will focus on the structure of the arguments themselves and the ways existing data are recruited to support them.

The health-oriented critics claim that informed consent is ineffective in achieving its primary goals. They generally make one of two points. First, patients do not understand or use the information they are given, and thus to require physicians to spend time disclosing information to patients constitutes a wasteful use of scarce health resources. Second, informed consent is actually deleterious to patients' health. Both arguments are rooted in a belief that patients are simply unable to deal with medical information in a matter that results in meaningful decisions.

Franz Ingelfinger, late editor of the *New England Journal of Medicine,* exemplified this approach in an editorial entitled "Informed (but Uneducated) Consent" (19). "The chances are remote," he noted, speaking in the research context, "that the subject really understands what he had consented to." Not only will the subject have difficulty comprehending the true import of discomforts and risks associated with any procedure, but "it is moreover quite unlikely that any patient-subject can see himself accurately within the broad context of the situation, to weigh the inconveniences and hazards that he will have to undergo against the improvements that the research project may bring to the management of his disease in general and to his own case in particular." Many research studies that purport to demonstrate poor patient understanding of relevant information are usually cited in support of such contentions.

One of the better studies reports the results of testing 50 patients "within an hour of their admission to . . . [a clinical research] Center and their consent interview with the physician-investigator" (20). All subjects had just consented to a clinical research project and had presumably read and had signed a consent form (22 percent of the subjects failed to read the form in its entirety). Of the subjects, 52 percent were judged to be adequately knowledgeable, based on their responses to a 19-item questionnaire. Only a minority had what the investigators defined as sufficient knowledge of the procedures (34 percent), the purpose (22 percent), and the risks (20 percent) of the study. In assessing this poor performance, the authors found problems with the format and content of the consent forms, the manner of presentation, and the circumstances in which the patient-subjects were situated.

This study suffered from the common defects of most investigations of patient or subject understanding. Oral disclosure was neither observed nor standardized, and the authors were forced to assume that the information whose comprehension they were measuring was actually conveyed, either in written form or in some unrecorded oral form. Furthermore, the ability to recall information, even a short time after a decision has been made, is not necessarily an indication of the understanding of the information at the time of the decision itself. The authors in this study were more sophisticated than most in pointing to multifactorial causes of poor understanding and in suggesting improvements in consent practices rather than totally rejecting the idea of informed consent.

Data of this sort, produced repeatedly by different research groups (see references) in [18]), are often used to support the argument that understanding *cannot* be achieved. Such statements are easily refuted by reference to studies of situations in which reasonable comprehension actually has been achieved (21–23). A sounder interpretation of all these studies might be that patients and subjects can attain a good level of understanding in many cases, but that several factors—including the manner in which disclosure is made as well as patients' limitations—may get in the way.

A variation on the Ingelfinger argument relies not so much on patients' noncomprehension as their proclivity to make decisions with little reference to the information they have. Fellner and Marshall, for example, studied decisions in kidney donors (a most atypical population) and claimed that the decision to donate or not was always made before any information was provided, usually on grounds irrelevant to the medical issues at hand (24). More typically, perhaps, a study of the effect of disclosure on contraceptive choice found that 93 percent of the patients reported having made up their minds before disclosure, and only 4 percent said the disclosure changed their decision (25).

Alternatively, it is argued that patients are so reliant on their physicians' advice that regardless of the information they receive, they will passively place the decision in their physician's hands. Even without such passive trust, some physicians have claimed that they can almost always get their patients to consent to any procedure they desire to perform—even in the research setting (26). If information is either not understood, or not considered in a patient's decision, the health-oriented critics maintain, it makes little sense to require physicians to provide it or hold them liable for failure to do so.

The second prong of the health-oriented critique concerns not only the waste of time and resources involved in an informed consent process but also the actual harm that might result from disclosure. Of course the courts, beginning with *Salgo* (as Katz notes), have had similar concerns, accounting for their deference to medical discretion, professional standards of disclosure, and the therapeutic privilege. A number of rather sensational case reports have purported to show instances when the disclosure of possible risks to patients led to untoward results, including cardiac problems, unjustified refusal of treatment, and death, either self-inflicted or as the result of the untreated disease (27–29). The conclusions drawn from these anecdotal accounts are that more patients are being harmed than helped by informed consent discussions. "I would propose," suggests one physician-author, "that we provide patients with reasonable explanations of what we feel is appropriate and not permit lawyers or administrators to set the rules" (28).

Few critics working from the health-oriented perspective make much more specific suggestions than this one as to what approach they would prefer to the current system. Implicit in many articles appears to be the wish that the legal requirements for informed consent would just go away, leaving physicians with the nearly total discretion they had in the days of "simple consent." In almost no case is any recognition given to the legitimate interest of patients in making their own decisions, participating in the decisionmaking process, or even knowingly ceding the right to make decisions to their medical caretakers. Insofar as the existence of competing interests and the impracticality of rolling back thirty years of case law and statutes is ignored, the health-oriented critique of informed consent has been a theoretical failure. The irony is, however, that even with weak empirical grounding and a monocular view of the world, this critique has had a substantial impact on many of the courts and legislatures that have struggled to shape legal rules to govern informed consent. The discretion retained by physicians in current law, as Katz has noted, results largely from the lawmakers' fears of constructing a system that might actually cause harm to patients, even though such fears may in fact be groundless.

7.3 The Interactionist Critique

The most original and provocative critique of informed consent rejects both autonomy and health as the ultimate goals. Robert Burt, in his book *Taking Care of Strangers*, has attempted to shift the focus of the debate away from the outcomes and toward the process (30). Burt's primary value in the doctor-patient interaction is respect for the humanity of each participant. In promoting this goal, Burt would reject the claims of both patient and physician advocates to dominance in the decisionmaking process. Dominance itself, in Burt's view, is incompatible with the kind of respect he is seeking to promote. His work is the only comprehensive effort so far to rethink the rationale for informed consent and to offer a carefully worked out alternative. His analysis, despite some problems with the implications he draws from it, warrants careful examination.

Burt begins with a thoroughgoing skepticism about efforts to enhance patient autonomy through the process of disclosure and consent. Truly autonomous decision making, he believes, is an impossibility. Human beings operate within social frameworks, and any decision made within a dyadic relationship, such as that between doctor and patient, cannot help but be influenced by what both parties bring to the interaction. Moreover, both doctor and patient will change as they come to know and begin to share each other's values. This process is more emotional than rational. The intense feelings generated in a relationship in which life and death are often at stake will frequently have a more potent impact on the participants than any position they reach as the result of purely cognitive processes.

The resistance to recognizing the mutuality that must dominate the decisionmaking process, Burt would say, stems from fear: fear of acknowledging the dependency and impotence that both parties share in the face of often irreversible natural forces; fear of the inherent uncertainty of their situation; fear of death. Doctors and patients alike attempt to master their fears by seeking complete control of the interpersonal scene. It is as if physician and patient are each saying to the other, "If I can master you and control this interaction in which we are engaged, then I can control anything. I will no longer be powerless and uncertain in the face of death."

If we are to humanize doctor-patient interactions, according to this view, we must transform this struggle for control into a collaborative effort to confront the participants' mutual fears. Doctor and patient could be encouraged or even compelled to talk with each other, in fact to negotiate with each other, respecting each other's independence and humanity. The law of informed consent can be a crucial tool in this process. Burt would compel such dialogue and negotiation by leaving all parties in doubt as to what the law requires of them. Since physicians could never be certain that anything they did effectively insulated them from suit, they would always be driven to ascertain patients' desires, work with them to shape a reasonable and mutually satisfactory plan of treatment, and in the process provide all the information patients want. Should a suit be brought after the fact, alleging that the physician had been negligent in the process, the case would be judged by a general standard of reasonableness, without predefined rules.

Burt's analysis has evoked considerable response, primarily from the legal profession. Most commentators have avoided criticizing his view of the emotional basis of the doctor-patient relationship and instead have targeted his proposed solution. Clearly, there would be immense legal difficulties in implementing Burt's scheme. Law works toward achieving certainty rather than uncertainty. A situation in which neither side could know with assurance the consequences of its behavior would strike many as unfair. In addition, it is difficult to imagine how that uncertainty might be maintained, that is, how one could prevent precedent from developing (e.g., in defining what constitutes a reasonable effort on the physician's part). It is almost impossible to envision how one might implement Burt's scheme.

Yet, Burt's contribution, elements of which have been echoed by Jay Katz, should not be overlooked (2, pp. 142–154). By emphasizing that the problem to be addressed is one of modifying interpersonal relationships, not formulating legal rules, Burt and Katz (in his more recent writing, 2) tear us away from the arguments over legal standards of disclosure and causation. They refocus our attention on the fact that the law is of dubious efficacy in regulating how people interact. It can establish the prerequisites for interaction of the desired type (as by requiring that a discussion about a patient's impending medical decision take place), but it is quite helpless to affect the tone or goodwill of the interaction.

7.4 A Synthetic Approach

We find it difficult to question the validity of much of what critics on all sides of the informed consent controversy have had to say. Like the autonomy-oriented commentators, we believe firmly in the importance of patients having the opportunity to participate in making medical decisions. That conclusion appeals to us on deontologic grounds—we take as fundamental the idea that patients should have the right to decide what happens to their bodies. On consequentialist grounds, our research, along with others', has suggested that patients are more likely to aid in their own care if they understand and have played a role in selecting the treatment they receive (4, pp. 378–374; 31, pp. 468–470).

On the other hand, like the health-oriented critics we recognize that whatever legal requirements are established to enforce the doctrine of informed consent should not so impede the delivery of medical care that instead of improving patients' well-being the doctrine actually causes patients harm. Thus, while we agree that steps need to be taken to encourage greater communication between physicians and patients, some proposals—including such punitive measures as a system of tort-fines that would be imposed whenever physicians are deficient in disclosing information—seem to us to have the potential for causing more harm than good. Physicians who are overly concerned about the possibility of being sued for what they say will say very little, at least spontaneously. The essential interactive nature of the physician-patient relationship will be lost, as physicians and patients glower at each other in suspicion. To save patient autonomy at the expense of destroying the very relationship that is essential for proper medical care is a Pyrrhic victory.

We part company with both autonomy- and health-oriented critics—at least from the more extreme members of each group—in our belief that the law of informed consent cannot univalently support either of these interests. To grant that the legal doctrine of informed consent compromises patient autonomy to some extent is not, as some would claim, to declare it worthless in that regard. There is little doubt that, however poorly it has been implemented to date, the slowly growing acceptance of the idea of informed consent among doctors and patients has led to substantially greater communication of information than occurred in the past. If the legal requirements have not gone as far as they might in stimulating communication, a major obstacle has been the concern that patients' health might be harmed thereby—hardly a meretricious motivation.

Similarly, although the law of informed consent makes physicians' lives more difficult and permits some patients to make bad health decisions, this price is not an unreasonable one to pay for the support of a value as important as the right of individual choice. The argument that informed consent simply does not work because patients do not understand or utilize the information they receive also does not vitiate the value of the idea of collaborative decision making. As noted above, some studies suggest that the decision-making process, properly carried out, can result in patients having a good understanding of the information disclosed. Even if a fair number of patients fail to understand or decline to make use of the information they receive, the idea of informed consent still has value in that it offers all patients the opportunity to participate in their care. Patients do and should have the right to reject that opportunity, either implicitly by ignoring the information provided, or explicitly by waiver, and it is wrong to deny them the choice. Thus, the fact that the idea of informed consent is something less in practice than it is in theory in no way suggests that it should be abandoned, even if it has certain costs in terms of medical time and effort.

The compromises that have been struck between the values of autonomy and of health, as detailed throughout this book, do not as a whole strike us as unreasonable ones. Although we might quarrel with one or another choice made by courts or legislatures, we do not share the apocalyptic visions of critics of both persuasions. In fact, the continuing attention paid to the nuances of the law of informed consent seems entirely misplaced. For the reasons so well described by the autonomy-oriented critics, and supported by empirical studies, the law has had surprisingly little impact on most doctor-patient interactions. It is unlikely that any legal rules can, by themselves, lead to very much additional alteration in physicians' practices without becoming so intrusive as to inhibit the effective provision of medical care.

How then can the idea of informed consent, with its vision of collaborative decision making between physicians and patients, be more nearly approximated in day-to-day medical care? We share the view of Burt and Katz that it certainly cannot be done without the cooperation of physicians (30, pp. 124–143; 2, pp. 228–229). This cooperation in turn can only be garnered if the medical profession can be weaned from its view of informed consent as a pernicious, alien doctrine imposed by a hostile legal system. More stringent legal rules are not the answer, since they will only evoke increased resistance from physicians, who after all still remain in control of both the content and tone of doctor-patient interactions. Yet, the medical profession will not accept informed consent unless their belief that it is incompatible with good medical care can be dispelled.

We believe this goal is attainable. The development of the law of informed consent has been premised on a set of irreconcilable conflicts between autonomy and health, and the extent of those conflicts has been greatly exaggerated. Whatever the divergences in theory, when it comes to the clinical setting, the principles of good medical care and informed consent, properly conceived, are not in opposition. For physician behavior to change, physicians must be persuaded of two conclusions: that (1) patients should have the right to participate in decision making, and (2) in fact, appropriate implementation of informed consent reinforces the doctor-patient dialogue that lies at the core of an effective therapeutic relationship, thus facilitating good medical care.

That many physicians now think otherwise is a function in part of their training about the relative rights and responsibilities of doctors and patients. (How physicians' beliefs might come to include the theories underlying the idea of informed consent is considered in some detail in the concluding section of this book—see Chapter 13.) Physicians' views have also been shaped significantly by their experiences with a species of informed consent (what we call in the next chapter the event model of informed consent) that in paying obeisance to the legal requirements wholly ignores the realities of clinical care. We demonstrate in the following chapter that this need not be the case.

References

1. Katz J: Informed consent—a fairy tale? Law's vision. *University of Pittsburgh Law Review* 39:137–174, 1977.

2. Katz J: *The Silent World of Doctor and Patient*. New York, Free Press, 1984.

3. Salgo v. Leland Stanford Jr. University Board of Trustees, 154 Cal. App.2d 560, 317 P.2d 170 (1957).

4. Lidz CW, Meisel A: Informed consent and the structure of medical care, in President's Commission for the Study of Ethical Problems in Medicine and Biomedical and Behavioral Research, *Making Health Care Decisions: The Ethical and Legal Implications of Informed Consent in the Patient-Practitioner Relationship.* Vol. 2, Appendices. Washington, D.C., U.S. Government Printing Office, 1982.

5. Lidz CW, Meisel A, Zerubavel E, et al.: *Informed Consent: A Study of Decisionmaking in Psychiatry.* New York, Guilford, 1984.

6. Harris L, and associates: Views of informed consent and decisionmaking: parallel surveys of physicians and the public, in President's Commission for the Study of Ethical Problems in Medicine and Biomedical and Behavioral Research, *Making Health Care Decisions: The Ethical and Legal Implications of Informed Consent in the Patient-Practitioner Relationship.* Vol. 2, Appendices. Washington, D.C., U.S. Government Printing Office, 1982.

7. Strull WM, Lo B, Charles G: Do patients want to participate in medical decisionmaking? *JAMA* 252:2990–2994, 1984.

8. Simpson RE: Informed consent: from disclosure to patient participation in medical decisionmaking. *Northwestern University Law Review* 76:172–207, 1981.

9. Rice N: Informed consent: the illusion of patient choice. *Emory Law Journal* 23:503–522, 1974.

10. Schneyer TJ: Informed consent and the danger of bias in the formation of medical disclosure practices. *Wisconsin Law Review* 1976:124–170.

11. Glass ES: Restructuring informed consent: legal therapy for the doctor-patient relationship. *Yale Law Journal* 79:1533–1576, 1970.

12. Riskin LL: Informed consent: looking for the action. *University of Illinois Law Forum* 1975:580–511.

13. Meisel A: The expansion of liability for medical accidents: from negligence to strict liability by way of informed consent. *Nebraska Law Review* 56:51–152, 1977.

14. Goldstein J: For Harold Lasswell: some reflections on human dignity, entrapment, informed consent, and the plea bargain. *Yale Law Journal* 84:683–703, 1975.

15. DiMatteo MR, DiNicola DD: *Achieving Patient Compliance: The Psychology of the Medical Practitioner's Role.* New York, Pergamon Press, 1982.

16. Janis IL: *Psychological Stress: Psychoanalytic and Behavioral Studies of Surgical Patients.* New York, Wiley, 1958.

17. President's Commission for the Study of Ethical Problems in Medicine and Biomedical and Behavioral Research: *Making Health Care Decisions: The Ethical and Legal Implications of Informed Consent in the Patient-Practitioner Relationship.* Vol. 1, *Report.* Washington, D.C., U.S. Government Printing Office, 1982.

18. Meisel A, Roth LH: Toward an informed discussion of informed consent: a review and critique of the empirical studies. *Arizona Law Review* 25:265–346, 1983.

19. Ingelfinger FJ: Informed (but uneducated) consent. *N Engl J Med* 287:465–466, 1972.

20. Schultz AL, Pardee GP, Ensinck JW: Are research subjects really informed? *West J Med* 123:76–80, 1975.

21. Woodward WE: Informed consent of volunteers: a direct measurement of comprehension and retention of information. *Clin Res* 27:248–252, 1979.

22. Bergler JH, Pennington AC, Metcalfe M, et al.: Informed consent: how much does the patient understand? *Clin Pharmacol Ther* 4:435–440, 1979.

23. Howard JM, DeMets D, BHAT Research Group: How informed is informed consent? The BHAT experience. *Controlled Clinical Trials* 2:287–303, 1981.

24. Fellner CH, Marshall JR: Kidney donors—the myth of informed consent. *Am J Psychiatry* 126:1245–1251, 1970.

25. Faden RR, Beauchamp TL: Decisionmaking and informed consent: a study of the impact of disclosed information. *Social Indicators Research* 7:314–336, 1980.

26. Beecher HK: Consent in clinical experimentation: myth and reality. *JAMA* 195:124–125, 1966.

27. Kaplan SR, Greenwald RA, Rogers AJ: Neglected aspects of informed consent. *N Engl J Med* 296:1127, 1977.

28. Katz RL: Informed consent—is it bad medicine? *West J Med* 126:426–428, 1977.

29. Patten BM, Stump W: Death related to informed consent. *Tex Med* 74:49:50, 1978.

30. Burt RA: *Taking Care of Strangers: The Rule of Law in Doctor-Patient Relations.* New York, Free Press, 1979.

31. Appelbaum PS, Roth LH: Treatment refusal in medical hospitals, in President's Commission for the Study of Ethical Problems in Medicine and Biomedical and Behavioral Research, *Making Health Care Decisions: The Ethical and Legal Implications of Informed Consent in the Patient-Practitioner Relationship*. Vol. 2, Appendices. Washington, D.C., U.S. Government Printing Office, 1982.

III

THE CLINICAL SETTING

8

Informed Consent in Practice

How can informed consent be integrated into the physician-patient relationship in a manner that is respectful of both the idea of informed consent and the imperatives of clinical care? A realistic answer to that question could, we believe, remove much of the resistance to the idea of informed consent that has been manifested by the medical profession to date. This chapter offers a practical procedural framework within which clinicians can operate to assist patients' decisions in a manner that meets both these desiderata.

8.1 Two Models

The interactions of physicians and patients in making decisions about medical treatment can be conceptualized in two ways. Decision making can be approached as an event that occurs at a single point in time: an event model. Alternatively, decision making can be viewed as a continuous element of the relationship between patients and their caregivers: a process model. The implications of these different ways of conceptualizing decisions about treatment are quite profound, since they are rooted in distinct visions of the relationship between physicians and patients.

The Event Model

A relatively simple paradigm is the basis of the event model of informed consent. A patient seeking medical care approaches a physician for assistance. After assessing the patient's condition, the physician reaches a diagnosis and formulates a recommended plan of treatment. The physician's conclusion and recommendations are presented to the patient along with information on the risks and benefits, and the possible alternatives and their risks and benefits. Weighing the available data, the patient reflects on the relative risks and benefits of each course of action and then makes the medically acceptable choice that most closely fits his or her particular values.

On the surface at least, this model conforms well to the legal requirements for informed consent. The model emphasizes the provision of full and accurate information to patients at the time of decision. Consent forms are often used for this purpose. In fact, the consent form can be said to be the central symbol of the event model. Patients' understanding, although desirable in the abstract, is less crucial to this model than is the provision of information. Once information is provided, patients make clear-cut choices about treatment, offering physicians straightforward guidance as to whether legally effective consent has been obtained, and treatment can proceed.

In the event model, decision making is temporally circumscribed. It begins when a physician makes recommendations with information and it ends with the patient's decision. Information that patients bring to this interaction, including previous communications from physicians, is considered outside the scope of the current decisionmaking event. Similarly, although patients are nominally free to change their minds about treatment, whatever occurs after the decision has been made is also irrelevant to the decision, unless one party or the other desires to reopen the issue by initiating another decisionmaking event.

The event model offers several advantages that give it favor in many medical settings, but it also offers reason for pause. On the positive side of the ledger, the event model is clearly preferable to more physician-dominated procedures, in which patients are offered little information and given no chance to participate in decision making. The event model, to its credit, provides patients with considerable information about their care and an opportunity to make choices.

Moreover, this model fits well with the contemporary arrangement of hospital, clinic, and office-based medical care. Most modern health-care facilities, both large medical centers and private offices, now break down care into a series of discrete, smaller tasks. Each of these tasks may be the responsibility of a different member of a health-care team. A receptionist obtains demographic and insurance information; a nurse elicits a chief complaint and measures some physiological parameters; a physician performs a physical examination and determines what additional data are needed; a variety of technicians conduct tests to provide the data. Even the responsibilities of physicians are subdivided by time (patients may be assigned to the doctor on call, rather than a personal physician) and specialty.

This differentiation of medical care functions has developed in response to the rapid growth of medical knowledge, and to economic pressures, which encourage minimization of the time spent with patients by the most highly salaried members of the team. Comparisons with assembly-line procedures in factories are unfair in some regards, but the underlying efficiency-based rationale is similar. The event model meets the needs of this differentiated system. Decision making can be assigned to a particular place ("Will you please see Ms. Smith in Room 7 at the end of the hall"), person ("I am Ms. Smith, Dr. Jones' nurse; I will read you the consent form, answer your questions, and get your consent"), and time ("We need to have you read and sign this now"). Obtaining the patient's consent need not be a concern before or after the assigned time, or for members of the team outside of whose responsibilities the task falls.

From the patient's point of view, too, the event model offers some advantages. There is little ambiguity about the roles of the members of the health-care team. The person who obtains consent is precisely identified. The time when a decision must be made is clearly demarcated. And patients may have a good idea, in the end, of just what they have consented to and when consent was obtained.

On the other hand, there are substantial problems with the event model. For one thing, it presumes that medical care conforms strictly to the paradigm outlined above—that is, that medical care involves a single decision, or small number of decisions, made at discrete points in time, when sufficient information is available. In fact, observational research on the structure of medical decision making (1, pp. 166–201; 2, pp. 336–339) suggests that it is rare for the care of a patient to involve only a single decision or for the needed information all to be available when a decision must be made. More commonly, treatment strategies evolve over time as additional information becomes available, including data from diagnostic tests and the results of previous empirical therapy. This situation is particularly common with chronic illnesses, but also applies to conditions of relatively recent onset whose etiology is unclear.

A fever of unknown origin offers a good example here. When a patient with fever and no localizing signs is admitted to a hospital, a diagnosis of the different possibilities will be constructed and a plan formulated to investigate each one. Each test will yield some amount of information. As the tests become increasingly invasive and present greater risks of their own, more and more difficult decisions have to be made about their value to the workup (3, pp. 3–19). In addition, indications may become stronger on empirical grounds for a trial of antibiotics, which itself entails risks of potential side effects and the possibility that the underlying cause of the fever will be obscured. There is no single decision to be made at a discrete point in time here as envisioned by the event model of decision making. Rather, multiple decisions must be made, often on a daily basis, as additional information becomes available. Adherence to the event model, with doctor and patient waiting for information to accumulate sufficient for a definitive decision, will leave the patient out of decision making altogether while the physician conducts the workup. And insofar as the evaluation may be difficult to separate from treatment (e.g., a trial of antibiotics is both diagnostic and therapeutic) and presents risks and benefits of its own, these decisions are precisely the kind in which patient involvement is anticipated by the idea of informed consent.

The event model may be problematic even in situations where only a single decision must be made, because of the model's assumption that the decision will be made at a discrete time. Evidence suggests that it is often extremely difficult to pinpoint exactly when medical decisions are made (1, pp. 202–231). Information often accumulates progressively, with each additional datum leading the doctor toward recommending a particular treatment option. The cumulative effect of the information obtained over time may be to make the final decision appear to be preordained when the decisionmaking event finally arrives. Neither doctor nor patient at that point may feel as though there is anything left to decide. If the patient has been excluded from the decisionmaking process until then, on the ground that the time for making a decision had not yet arrived, the goal of patient participation that underlies the idea of informed consent will be subverted.

Furthermore, the event model appears to be structured in the worst possible way as far as facilitating patients' being informed. Educators have long known that the provision of information repetitively over a sustained period results in better understanding and better retention than one exposure. Information is more effectively assimilated when patients are at relative ease than at times of stress. The event model encourages education of patients on one occasion, with little opportunity for reflection and integration of the information into the patients' underlying scheme of values. And this is done at a time—given that a decision must be made imminently—when patients' anxiety is likely to be at a peak. Thus, the event model inhibits precisely the kind of understanding participation on which the idea (although perhaps not the legal doctrine) of informed consent is based. Numerous studies show poor patient understanding and limited retention of information provided in physician disclosures and consent forms. (See Chapter 9.) This problem is at least in part a reflection of the failure of the educational function in an event model.

Physicians sense these deficiencies in the event model, even as they employ it because it makes their lives easier in some respects. Their recognition that patients are not truly participating in decision making, or participating with limited understanding, contributes to their rejection of the idea of informed consent. It seems farcical to spend time talking with patients in detail about some

of the least important decisions that need to be made—in the sense
of having been preordained by other events—when the earlier,
more influential decisions have been made by physicians alone. It
seems a waste of time to present patients with elaborate consent
forms when they so rarely seem to understand the information
critical to a decision. In short, the event model perpetuates a view
of informed consent as something detached from the unique
rhythm of the clinical setting— something imposed on medicine
by an uncomprehending legal system.

These considerations suggest that a model of decision making
is needed that recognizes both the temporal complexity of medical
decisions and patients' pedagogic needs. Such an approach is found
in the "process model" of decision making and consent.

The Process Model

In contrast to the event model, the process model of informed
consent is based on the assumption that medical decision making
is a continuous process, and the exchange of information must take
place throughout the course of the physician-patient relationship.
We use the term exchange, implying a two-way transfer of information, deliberately. To facilitate patient participation in decision
making, physicians need to disclose information to patients about
recommended and alternative diagnostic and therapeutic approaches, as it becomes available. And patients need to discuss
their concerns with their physicians—including their understanding
of the choices that face them, questions they may have, and the
values they particularly want reflected in their medical care.

We refer to the process of interchange of information as mutual
monitoring, because it permits each party to monitor the factors
that are entering into the other's thinking at any given time. Such
monitoring requires sensitivity on the part of both physicians and
patients. Physicians need to offer information in an appropriate
fashion, so as to educate, not confuse, patients. This model does
not imply stream-of-consciousness revelations by physicians. Patients should not be greeted at the initial encounter, for example,
with a terrifying list of potential diagnoses, including remote and
often fatal possibilities. Such disclosure is likely to immobilize
rather than illuminate. Instead, information that is relevant to the

next necessary decision should be offered to patients as it is developed. (The differentiation of disclosure according to the phase of treatment will be described below.)

Patients, too, have an active role to play in the process model, in comparison with their relatively passive part in the event model. Their role expands in three directions. First, it is anticipated that they will interact with their physicians as information is provided, asking questions, clarifying ambiguities, helping physicians understand the values they choose to promote. Second, patients will be faced with an increased number of choices. Finally, since the selection of a course of treatment can usually be modified as mutual monitoring takes place, patients have a responsibility to provide feedback to physicians about the effect of treatment on the target symptoms and their degree of satisfaction with regard to their individual goals and values.

The advantages of a process model are substantial. It conforms as much to the requirements of the legal doctrine as the event model does, and simultaneously promotes the underlying idea of informed consent. Patients are brought actively into the decision-making process in a manner that encourages their knowing participation. They receive information, over time, in a fashion that allows it to be contemplated, shared, and assimilated. And because patients participate in the stream of preliminary decisions that may, in effect, predetermine the outcome, they are more effectively included in the ultimate decision.

Additional benefits come from the enhanced alliance between physicians and patients envisioned by the process model. Patients may begin to perceive that treatment decisions are their own, not just their physicians'. As patients develop greater identification with the decision and an increased ability to understand what treatment entails, compliance may be improved. Further, patients who see themselves as intimately involved in medical decision making may be less likely to sue alleging malpractice; suits alleging lack of informed consent should become particularly rare.

Finally, and perhaps most importantly, the process model, in reflecting the realities of medical care, should serve to make the idea of informed consent meaningful to physicians. The disclosure and consent process is not divorced from the real decisions that need to be made. To be sure, the process model demands of physicians more substantial efforts to integrate patients' views into the decisions that need to be made but in contrast to the event model, there will be a clear purpose to the whole effort. Patients and doctors will work together in a process that is meaningful, not merely formal.

As with all approaches, there are also disadvantages. Physicians are not accustomed to discussing their thoughts and information with patients except when an event-model type of decision needs to be made. Substantial retraining might be required before most physicians could function comfortably in the process model. Similarly, patients who are accustomed—whatever their degree of frustration—to functioning passively in doctor-patient relationships will have to be reeducated about their new role. Both kinds of reeducation require time and money and could meet with resistance. The kind of interaction envisioned will also consume additional time, although perhaps not as much as many practitioners might fear. Hospital schedules and the organization of the average physician's day may have to be restructured to some extent.

Do the advantages outweigh the disadvantages? We believe they do. Many of the relative benefits and costs ought to be measurable in appropriately designed studies. Although there are significant a priori reasons to endorse a process model, they have yet to be empirically substantiated.

8.2 The Stages of Treatment in the Process Model

The basic principle of the process model is that patients should be able to participate in decision making in every phase of care. Such participation should be a continual facet of all interactions, woven into the very fabric of the doctor-patient relationship. How this principle works in practice may be envisioned most easily by examining its operation through the stages of patient care. These stages can be characterized by the five primary tasks they address: establishing the relationship, defining the problem, ascertaining the goals of treatment, selecting a therapeutic plan, and follow-up. Of course, the tasks do not always proceed in this order, and several may be addressed simultaneously. Each requires physicians to provide patients with information relating to a key question so that they may make appropriate decisions.

Establishing the Relationship

The key question for patients when the relationship with a physician is first established is, Do I want to entrust my care to this person? This question is not always asked or answered definitively at the very beginning. If patient and physician first meet as the patient lies on a stretcher in an emergency room writhing in pain, treatment ordinarily will proceed with minimal attention by the patient to the question of whether this is the appropriate physician. Even in this setting, however, the physician must establish to the patient's satisfaction a basis for authority to treat. This may involve a statement as simple as, "I am Dr. Jones, the physician on call here tonight, and I have responsibility for all patients admitted." In an emergency setting, patients in need of care are likely to accept this information as sufficient. When making decisions at greater leisure, of course, patients may desire additional information before entrusting their care to a particular physician. They may want to know about the physician's specialty, particular interests and skills, and any unique aspects of the relationship (e.g., the physician will nominally be in charge, but actual care will be rendered by a junior associate).

The establishment of a relationship, though rarely explicitly considered by practitioners, is a constant element of medical care. In outpatient settings, where patients have a variety of options for health care, the process of evaluating a physician often proceeds as a matter of course, with physicians providing the necessary information without even being aware of doing so. In hospital care, however, where patients are perceived as having limited choices as to who undertakes their treatment, physicians often neglect to provide the information patients need for deciding to be cared for or not by a given physician.

The problem is complicated by the multiplicity of persons involved in inpatient care: attending physicians, house officers, consultants, technicians, nurses, social workers, and others. Patients are often least clear about consultants—who they are and why they should be allowed to participate in care. Consultants are frequently senior physicians, accustomed to being recognized in the hospital. They will often simply walk into a room, give their name, and begin an examination. Patients are understandably bewildered, not knowing why the examination is being conducted or who ordered it. They do not know whether the consultant is someone who can present new information to them or will make treatment decisions. The ambiguities in this situation are easy to clarify, with a simple statement such as, "Your doctor, Dr. Jones, asked me to come in and take a look at your eyes because I am a specialist in ophthalmology; I will be reporting my findings to him, and he will decide whether further action is needed." Yet, few physicians take the time to do so.

The way the doctor-patient relationship is established is crucial to all that follows in two senses. First, of course, if the patient declines to go any further with the relationship, no treatment will ensue. More subtly, the establishment of the relationship sets the tone for all subsequent treatment decisions. If physicians communicate to patients that they have little or no appropriate role in deciding whether a particular physician should undertake their care, patients are likely to assume a fortiori that they have even less chance of influencing the treatment decisions that follow. On the other hand, physicians who indicate to patients that they have a right to know who their physician is, and why he or she should be allowed to proceed with their care, signal that patients' participation will be welcome in subsequent treatment decisions.

Defining the Problem

The second key question is, What dysfunction will be the focus of treatment? Physicians often assume that this issue is purely technical. Researchers have demonstrated, however, that most medical problems are defined by a complex negotiation between physicians and patients (4, pp. 135–158; 5). Physicians who ignore patients' definitions of their problems will often end up with dissatisfied and resistant patients. To the degree that patients are committed to definitions of their problems and thus to particular treatment approaches, their inclinations to follow through with treatment are likely to be substantially greater (6, pp. 55–58). An example was reported by a physician who was afflicted by a syndrome that resulted in progressive blindness (7). From the treating physicians' point of view the problem to be addressed was the underlying pathology, for which little could be done. The patient-physician, however, defined his problem more broadly as learning how to cope with his failing eyesight. Having never discussed the patient's formulation of his problem, his physicians felt they had little to offer and retreated in the face of the inexorable progression of his illness. This procedure left him feeling embittered and abandoned. Ironically, the treating physicians had a great deal to offer in terms of helping the patient adjust to his diminished sight, suggesting devices for coping with lessened vision, and referring the patient to other caregivers who might be of additional help. Their failure to grasp this fact vitiated their potential to help. This sad ships-passing-in-the-night phenomenon occurs when patients and physicians have entirely different formulations of the problem to be treated.

Facilitating patients' participation at this phase means rejecting what has been called the high physician control style of patient care (8, 9). Typically, physicians employing this style begin by asking patients to describe their problems. Patients, perceiving difficulties in holding such physicians' attention, respond with brief accounts. Physicians then initiate long series of questions dealing with the patients' current symptoms and histories. A physical examination will usually ensue, sometimes accompanied by blood, radiographic, or other tests. Finally, with the data all collected, physicians announce the nature of the problem to their patients and order appropriate treatment. Physicians may ask if patients have any questions, but patients, recognizing that the interaction is about to be ended, will either reply in the negative or ask a brief question, often focused on the details of the therapeutic regimen. Patients never have a chance to define the problem in their own terms. Although in some sense a caricature, this description is not markedly different from those reported in several empirical studies (8,9).

In contrast, physicians operating under a process model of informed consent will encourage patients to participate actively in defining their problems. Since many patients have been socialized to passivity in doctor-patient relationships, physicians may need to ask open-ended questions and indicate their interest in complete responses. A recognition that patients are more likely to be disturbed by interferences with their daily lives than by underlying pathologic processes will help physicians to inquire appropriately. The ultimate, negotiated definition of the problem cannot ignore the need to address the pathology, but it must also take into account those results of the disease process that trouble patients the most.

Ascertaining the Goals of Treatment

Agreement between doctors and patients about the nature of the problem must be followed by consensus about the goals of treatment. Here the question for the patient is, What are the reasonable goals of therapy for the problem we have defined? Put somewhat differently, patients and physicians must collaborate at this point in defining the probable health career of the patient. Patients often have unrealistic expectations about their careers in the health system, in part because many conceptualize medical treatment with models drawn from surgery or the treatment of acute infectious diseases. They may expect to be cured of their illnesses and may assume that treatment that does not meet that expectation is a failure. Moreover, they may expect to be cured without much active effort on their part. This assumption is one source of the documented difficulty in obtaining patient compliance, particularly with treatments involving alteration of lifestyle (6).

Patients with chronic disorders often have particular difficulty understanding what constitute reasonable goals (10). For example, patients with chronic cardiac disorders may see their problem as recurring attacks of a lingering illness. They may believe that if only the doctor could find the proper medication or dosage, their problems would be cured. Patients with severe congestive heart failure may expect to go back to blue-collar jobs as soon as they "get well."

Patients with unrealistic goals for the future cannot engage in a a meaningful assessment of the risks and benefits of a proposed treatment. A procedure with substantial risks, such as coronary artery bypass surgery, might be a reasonable choice for a patient who expects substantial restoration of functioning, i.e., for whom the anticipated benefits are commensurate with the risks. If, however, the patient's heart muscle is already sufficiently damaged that restored blood flow is unlikely to bring improved functioning, the risks of surgery may not be worth taking. A patient who mistakes either situation for the other cannot make an informed decision. Thus, physicians must ensure that patients have an accurate understanding of the reasonable goals of treatment. Physicians should monitor patients' expectations and present sufficient information to correct distortions. Of course, sensitivity is required, since it is always desirable to maintain some degree of hope, either for a benign course or merely for maximal efforts to alleviate pain. Even when treatment can provide very little improvement in the patient's health, the physician should attempt to present the patient with a new goal to be achieved in treatment. What the patient chooses to do next should always seem important.

Physicians have not always made an effort to insure that patients' goals are realistic, particularly when doing so meant disclosure of patients' diagnoses and prognoses. Katz has pointed to Hippocrates' suggestions to physicians.

> Perform calmly and adroitly, concealing most things from the patient while you are attending him. Give necessary orders with cheerfulness and serenity, turning his attention away from what is being done to him . . . revealing nothing of the patient's future or present condition (11, p. 4).

Recently, there has been a strong movement toward more open disclosure. A study for the President's Commission on Ethical Problems in Medicine found substantial majorities of both physicians and patients in favor of disclosure of information such as a diagnosis of cancer (12). Research findings show that open disclosure to cancer patients leaves them with substantially less anxiety and depression (13).

In talking with cancer patients, we have found that they have two major complaints about their relationships with their physicians: first, that they were not being told enough, second, that they were given information in an insensitive manner. Their angriest feelings are toward physicians who told them that they would die within a specified period of time. By focusing on dying rather than on the fact that a patient might live for quite a while yet, the physician seemed to these patients to be removing any positive future. It is possible to tell a patient who has had an auto accident that resulted in a damaged spinal cord, "With work, you will be able to get around in a wheelchair and do a lot for yourself," rather than "You will never walk again." Receiving bad news is different from being left without anything to live for.

The process of negotiating goals of treatment will vary with the particular situation of each patient, but some constants exist. Physicians will need to begin by eliciting patients' goals, which necessarily will relate to their views of their illness and its likely outcome. In one form or another, the physician asks, "What were you hoping we could do for you?" and explores the basis for those expectations. When they are incongruent with reasonable medical outcomes, patients must be made aware of the divergence and more realistic goals suggested.

Sometimes, of course, patients will endorse a set of goals that are different from but no less achievable than the physician's. This may relate to differing perceptions of the nature of illness, with patients, for example, desiring relief of their most prominent symptoms (e.g., inability to sleep at night), while physicians focus on the underlying pathology (e.g., congestive heart failure). Alternatively, patients may be more or less aggressive than physicians depending on the degree of discomfort or disability they experience. Patients are often unaware of the possibilities of progression involved in a condition. Negotiation of a common set of goals thus requires the sharing of information by both parties as to their concerns and hopes. It is reciprocally related to the process of selecting appropriate treatment, since the selection of goals will often depend on the relative attractiveness of the methods by which they can be achieved.

Selecting an Approach to Treatment

Once the goals of treatment have been defined, patients and physicians must reach a decision on how to achieve them. The key question here for patients is, What treatment will present the best possible balance of risks and benefits? This aspect of treatment initiation generally attracts the most attention, although as we have seen, effective participation by patients in this phase is heavily dependent on what has already transpired between them and their physicians.

The disclosure required here is determined in part by the legal requirements for informed consent. That is, physicians must address the nature, purpose, risks, and benefits of treatment, along with the alternatives and their risks and benefits. Much of the required disclosure has been delineated earlier in this book. There are some additional concerns addressed here about disclosure of risks and alternatives and the timing of the discussions.

The difficulty in specifying exactly which risks should be disclosed has been noted. Common sense about what information patients need in order to make truly knowledgeable decisions is probably the physician's best guide. In addition, to encourage patients to reflect on their options, physicians may have to go beyond the narrow requirements of the law. The term risks may be somewhat limiting in its connotations here—many of the negative aspects of a particular treatment are not risks but certainties. Abdominal surgery, for example, always leaves patients with some degree of incisional pain and in need of a period of bed rest followed by a longer period of diminished activity. An adequate review of the predictable outcomes of surgery, including negative ones, should include coverage of the discomforts patients are certain to endure. Many jurisdictions exclude such so-called commonly known risks from the requirements for disclosure, but they may play a major role in patients' decisions. It is easy to see why a busy parent of young children might opt for a procedure with a shorter recuperation than for an alternative that involves prolonged bed rest, whatever its other advantages.

Disclosure and the discussion of alternatives raise important questions about the degree of neutrality to be sought by physicians. Neutrality may involve both values and opinions. Values describe deeply held beliefs—often religious and moral—or personal philosophies. There are some situations in which almost everyone would agree that physicians' own values ought to play no role in the decisionmaking process. For example, physicians' beliefs about the morality of elective abortions should not influence what they tell patients considering such procedures. (Physicians opposed to abortion on religious or other grounds obviously may refer a patient elsewhere rather than undertaking the procedure themselves.) At the other end of the spectrum, there may be occasions when patients invite physicians to share their values. For example, a patient dying of cancer may ask, "Doc, if it were you, would you go through with another course of chemotherapy on the chance that you'd get three months to live?" These situations are often sensitive. Patients may ask such questions in order to acquire ammunition for disputes with family members, or, unable to decide, may find some comfort in rejecting physicians' advice. Nevertheless, with a proper appreciation for the delicacy of the clinical setting, physicians can legitimately make their values known, especially when invited to do so.

Values may play another role in the discussion of alternatives. In many situations, patients may lack a clear sense of how particular treatments relate to values they hold dear. Physicians, because they deal with certain situations routinely, have sometimes thought more extensively about the religious, moral, or emotional issues involved, or are familiar with the typical reactions of other patients. When patients appear not to have recognized the implications of the choices they face, physicians might offer guidance by pointing out the values involved.

The difficulties that can arise without such guidance were illuminated by observations of decisions in a psychiatric clinic (1, pp. 128–129). A county mental health department had asked all hospitals treating psychiatric patients to pass on certain types of personal information, including patients' names, in order better to track utilization of health facilities in the county. The administration of one psychiatric facility decided that automatic release of this information would be a violation of patients' right to privacy and that they would allow release only with patients' consent. Clinicians staffing the admissions unit were instructed that the decision was completely a matter of patients' discretion.

In general, patients did whatever the clinician suggested, even though clinicians tried to keep from making patients' decisions for them. If a clinician said, "The county likes us to send information about people who consent; do you mind?" patients readily agreed. If a clinician suggested that it might be unfair to send such information, patients quickly denied permission. Some clinicians followed their instructions to the letter as follows:

Clinician:	Now one more thing. We send the county information about patients for statistics. If you don't want us to, you have the right to refuse to permit us to send any information about you. Write here [pointing] "O.K." or not.
Patient:	[didn't seem to understand]
Clinician:	If you don't want to, you can say no. It is up to you.
Patient:	[hesitating] I don't see any reason why I wouldn't want the county to know.
Clinician:	If you don't want to, you can write that there.
Patient:	I don't understand.
Clinician:	What don't you understand?
Patient:	You want me to choose whether to send this information to the county?
Clinician:	Yes.
Patient:	Will that benefit the hospital?
Clinician:	Don't worry about the hospital. I don't want to influence you. This is your decision.

The patient eventually agreed to release the information but later told the interviewer, "Did you see me? I was so confused about the thing about the county. I thought, 'Now if I don't let them release the information, will they make me an involuntary patient or is it that if you want a job with them that they will have records on it?' I was so confused." Another patient wondered whether releasing the information would interfere with her getting a county job later, but her husband prevailed, suggesting that the county might later hold it against her that she had refused to release the information when she applied for a job.

   In general, these patients did not have the requisite background knowledge to assess what values were at stake. Part of this difficulty was a lack of purely factual information. Many chronic psychiatric patients equated the county with its welfare component, and many working-class patients knew it mostly as a source of jobs. The concept of a bureaucracy trying to control health costs and needing information to do so was alien to them. Furthermore, the abstract value of a right to privacy, when the release of the information could not be shown to do any immediate harm, was difficult for them to comprehend. This is not to say, of course, that they had no feelings about these issues, merely that without an explanation of their relevance to the current decision they were lost. In some situations, part of an adequate informed consent process is a review with the patient of what values are at stake. One cannot take it for granted that patients will consider the issue fully without explanation.

In contrast to values, physicians' opinions relate to the conclusions they draw from medical facts, although it is impossible for a physician to form opinions without some influence from an underlying set of values. Some have concluded that the idea of informed consent, with its heavy emphasis on patient autonomy, obliges physicians to act solely as technical consultants (14, p. 382). That is, physicians should provide information about the risks and benefits of the alternative treatments, then retire from the scene to allow patients to decide. In this model, physicians function like the television weather reporter who provides an objective forecast and then allows the viewer to decide whether a 40 percent chance of rain warrants cancellation of the Fourth of July picnic (15).

In the doctor-patient relationship, we believe this view is short-sighted. Ostensibly, for the sake of promoting autonomy, patients would be deprived of some of the most important information they may need. One of the most valuable skills physicians have to offer is the ability to integrate a large body of information about risks and benefits and arrive at appropriate recommendations. Some patients may wish to accept a physician's recommendation with little further reflection (16). Other patients will view physicians' suggestions as another piece of evidence—not necessarily a decisive one—to be considered. Although too strongly stated recommendations from physicians may overwhelm some patients' independence, there is also a risk that patients will misinterpret physicians' silence to mean that they believe all treatment options are equally desirable. Patients deserve a judicious recommendation—especially when requested—as an important part of the decisionmaking process.

In choosing the approach to treatment, another important issue is the temporal relationship between the selection of a treatment approach and the actual initiation of treatment—particularly when therapy is focused on a single major procedure as in most surgery.

By the time patients have psychologically prepared themselves for surgery, discussed it with family and friends, arranged their schedules to accommodate it, and checked into the hospital for two days of preliminary tests, they are clearly committed to having the operation. The decision has already been definitively made, at least from the patients' psychological perspective. They are hardly in a good position to make up their minds about whether or not to go through with a procedure to which they are already deeply committed. Consent obtained at this point is *pro forma*. Deferring serious discussion of treatment options to this time effectively deprives patients of a meaningful opportunity for decision making. At the same time, physicians who have followed the process model and already obtained patients' consent offer little or no additional benefit to their patients by reviewing the entire discussion. The same is true in the case of patients for whom surgery was not definitively contemplated prior to admission and who are kept informed about their course of treatment and diagnostic procedures throughout the period of hospitalization. In other words, patients who are well-informed and included in the decisionmaking process as it unfolds do not need a stylized consent procedure at the eleventh hour before surgery. In current practice, disclosure (often accompanied by the signing of a consent form) just prior to surgery, invasive diagnostic tests, electroconvulsive therapy, and similar procedures is routine. In fact, these discussions are often the only time that any systematic disclosure takes place. Although at this point the physician may usefully review the experiences the patient will have and offer to answer questions, serious consideration of whether or not to undertake surgery must take place at an earlier time (17,18).

Follow-up

Occasionally, treatment will be a one-time event—for example, the excision of a mole. More usually, once a course of treatment is selected and implemented, the effectiveness of the interventions must be evaluated and treatment modified accordingly. This is particularly true in the treatment of chronic illnesses, in which long-term doctor-patient relationships are the norm. Under the event model of decision making, the follow-up period is of little concern, unless a new event looms at some point in the future, when renewed interaction between physician and patient will be required. From the perspective of the process model this position looks naive, since it is recognized that new information is continuously becoming available and decisions always being made. The key question for patients at this stage is, Where do I stand relative to the decisions that were made when treatment was initiated?

At follow-up sessions, physicians must naturally elicit from patients the facts relevant to their conditions and treatment that have developed since the last interaction. This work is only half of the process of mutual monitoring that should take place. Physicians, too, must share information. They need to review the definition of the problem, the goals, and the treatment approaches that were decided upon previously, and insure that patients continue to share their understanding of these items. Patients' common reluctance to ask questions or admit to confusion means that physicians must take the initiative in exploring patients' understanding. A change in patient (or physician) perceptions may require renegotiation of one or more issues. In addition, physicians should detail the existence, import, and impact on the previous agreements of any new data.

Empirical studies suggest that physicians rarely follow this model. One study showed that less than five percent of a typical medical encounter period (less than one minute out of twenty) was spent by physicians in providing information to patients (19). Physicians are simply unaccustomed to explaining to patients the issues involved in making treatment decisions. Yet, without mutual monitoring, there is good reason to believe that mutual understanding between physicians and patients will rapidly dissipate.

Even assuming that complete understanding by both parties is achieved during the initial encounter, patients' views of illness and treatment do not remain static. They continue to ruminate on what they know. This continuous reordering of knowledge is one of the human mind's strongest and most creative features, and also the basis for a great deal of misunderstanding between physicians and patients. Each new event, such as the development of side effects from medication, and each new comment from physicians, family, or friends becomes an occasion to rethink and reconsider what is already known. This tendency is increased by the structure of modern health-care delivery. With a team of people (and sometimes three shifts of teams) engaged in the delivery of clinic and hospital care to a single patient, patients are likely to hear different and often conflicting information.

New information is not a necessary stimulus to patients' reconceptualization of treatment. Patients use cognitive processes like that which psychologists call *cognitive dissonance reduction* to reorganize and rethink their knowledge about treatment, even in the absence of new data. In reducing cognitive dissonance, patients try to build relatively simple cognitive fields that support the decisions that have already been made. Observational researchers have found, for example, that patients had trouble understanding that a medication given to relieve the side effects of another drug might have side effects of its own. Patients reduced the complexity of the information by reclassifying medications into those that caused side effects and those that relieved them. Thus, when they developed new side effects, they had trouble understanding why the doctor might want to lower the dose of the drug they saw as the medication that relieved side effects (1, pp. 278–279).

It is evident that an adequate decisionmaking process must include continual monitoring of patients' understanding. Sometimes exploration of patients' views will reveal a need to renegotiate some previously agreed-on aspect of treatment. Sometimes repetition or, in the light of new information, modification of the initial disclosure is required. Without repetition, the knowledge initially produced from disclosure can dissipate. If the repetition entails nothing more than the same words and phrases, it is unlikely that either patients or physicians will take them seriously. A good example of this type of disclosure is when airplane flight attendants provide information about safety. Because the presentation has become an empty ritual to flight attendants and passengers alike, neither party pays much attention to it after the first few times. The result is no new learning and no reinforcement of what was learned previously, so that learning quickly decays. Such a one-time learning process is particularly problematic in medicine, where the issues are continually changing, and what patients need to know may be somewhat different each time physicians and

patients meet. Thus, physicians are continually challenged to remain flexible in their approaches to discussions with patients, to
individualize disclosure to particular patients' needs and concerns,
and to avoid sterile repetition.

Another issue arises in the follow-up of patients who have, as
most patients do to some degree, become dependent on their caregivers and, now that they are recovering, harbor a sense of discomfort about that dependency. They may be unable or unwilling
to participate or collaborate in making decisions about their care.
They may attempt to reject their physicians' advice as a means of
reestablishing control. (The issues involved in patients' rejection
of treatment recommendations are discussed in detail in Chapter
10.) The process model of consent can help such patients to establish, maintain, or regain a sense of control without severing the
therapeutic relationship. Physicians can provide information about
the expected future course of the medical problem and help patients to integrate that information with their previous understanding of their medical careers. Emphasis should be placed on patients'
responsibility to manage their disorders, without giving the impression of abandonment by physicians. Thus, the continuing connection between physician and patient can be employed to confirm
patients' sense of autonomy.

Conclusion

The process model of medical decision making we have described
is in many ways an ideal. Few physicians and patients will be able
to fulfill the aspirations of the model in its entirety. Sometimes
time or economic pressures will intrude, and sometimes one or
both parties will choose to play a dominant or submissive role in
the relationship. But seen as an ideal, the process model provides
a goal concerned physicians and patients can strive for. It is the
concrete embodiment of the idea of informed consent, and the
logical extension of the ethical and legal theories from which that
idea developed. Further, in providing a model of informed consent
that conforms to the realities of clinical medicine, the process
model replaces the artificialities of the event model with meaningful and realistic procedures. With this approach, informed consent is no longer the farce or myth its physician critics have accused

it of being. It becomes an important and integral part of the doctor-patient relationship.

References

1. Lidz C, Meisel A, Zerubavel E, et al.: *Informed Consent: A Study of Decisionmaking in Psychiatry*. New York, Guilford, 1983.

2. Lidz CW, Meisel A: Informed consent and the structure of medical care, in President's Commission for the Study of Ethical Problems in Medicine and Biomedical and Behavioral Research, *Making Health Care Decisions: The Ethical and Legal Implications of Informed Consent in the Patient-Practitioner Relationship*. Vol. 2, Appendices. Washington, D.C., U.S. Government Printing Office, 1982.

3. Bursztajn H, Feinbloom RI, Hamm RM, Brodsky A: *Medical Choices, Medical Chances: How Patients, Families, and Physicians Can Cope with Uncertainty*. New York, Delacorte Press, 1981.

4. See Fisher S: Doctor Talk/Patient Talk: How Treatment Decisions Are Negotiated in Doctor-Patient Communication, in Fisher S, Todd A (eds.): *The Social Organization of Doctor-Patient Communication*. New York, Center for Applied Linguistics, 1983.

5. Eisenthal S, Emery R, Lazare A, et al.: "Adherence" and the negotiated approach to patienthood. *Arch Gen Psychiatry* 36:393–398, 1979.

6. DiMatteo MR, DiNicola DD: *Achieving Patient Compliance: The Psychology of the Medical Practitioner's Role*. New York, Pergamon, 1982.

7. Stetten D: Coping with blindness. *N Engl J Med* 305:458–460.

8. Platt FW, McMath JC: Clinical hypocompetence: the interview. *Ann Intern Med* 91:898–902, 1979.

9. Frankel RM: Talking in interviews: a dispreference for patient-initiated questions in physician-patient encounters, in Psathas G (ed.), *Interaction Competence*. New York, Irvington, 1983.

10. Lidz CW, Meisel A, Munetz M: Chronic disease: the sick role and informed consent. *Culture, Medicine and Psychiatry* 9:1–17, 1985.

11. Katz J: *The Silent World of Doctor and Patient*. New York, Free Press, 1984.

12. Harris L, and associates: Views of informed consent and decisionmaking: parallel surveys of physicians and the public, in President's Commission for the Study of Ethical Problems in Medicine and Biomedical and Behavioral Research, *Making Health Care Decisions: The Ethical and Legal Implications of Informed Consent in the Patient-Practitioner Relationship*. Vol. 2, *Appendices*. Washington, D.C., U.S. Government Printing Office, 1982.

13. Gerle B, Lundin G, Sandblom P: The patient with inoperable cancer from the psychiatric and social standpoint. *Cancer* 13:1206–1217, 1960.

14. Freidson E: *The Profession of Medicine*. New York, Dodd, Mead, 1970.

15. Lidz CW: The weather report model of informed consent: problems in preserving patient voluntariness. *Bull Am Acad Psychiatry Law* 8:152–160, 1980.

16. Ingelfinger FJ: Arrogance. *N Engl J Med* 303:1507–1511, 1980.

17. Langer EJ, Janis IL, Wolfer JA: Reduction of psychological stress in surgical patients. *J Experimental Soc Psychol* 11:155–165, 1975.

18. Vernon DTA: Information seeking in a natural stress situation. *J Applied Psychol* 55:359–363, 1971.

19. Waitzkin H: Doctor-patient communication: clinical implications of social scientific research. *JAMA* 252:2441–2446, 1984.

9

Consent Forms

The previous chapter described some of the problems of an event model of informed consent. The consent form was held up as the primary symbol of that model, and one might expect consideration of consent forms to consist mainly of warnings and injunctions against them. Unfortunately, the matter is not that simple.

In a number of situations, both practical and theoretical, consent forms are sometimes necessary. Most significantly, treatment facilities such as hospitals and clinics often require them. In certain circumstances, getting a consent form signed may be in the best interests of the physician-patient relationship. Moreover, in several jurisdictions, if a suit alleges lack of informed consent, there may be some advantages for a physician who has obtained the patient's signature on a written form. Finally, in the United States it is virtually impossible to conduct any government funded research in which there is more than minimal risk to subjects without consent forms. In fact, it is difficult to do any kind of substantial biomedical or behavioral research with human subjects without having to deal with consent forms in some way.

9.1 The Legal Status of Consent Forms

Consent forms are used routinely in both treatment and research settings, but there is considerable conflict about what purposes they are intended to serve. Two major purposes have been proposed. First, many attorneys, hospital administrators, physicians, and patients see consent forms primarily as protecting physicians and medical facilities from liability (1). This reason has become the dominant one, despite the fact that they may actually provide very little legal protection. Second, consent forms can be seen as part of the process of physicians educating patients about the proposed treatment (2). The pattern of use of consent forms will vary according to which model is adopted.

The history of the use of consent forms is unclear. What we now call a consent form probably evolved from the simple release of liability, a common legal document in hospital treatment, in which patients acknowledge that they agree to the proposed medical procedures and will not hold physicians liable for any ill effects resulting from their performance. Indeed some simple consent forms are still entitled "Release of Liability" or "Release." The modern consent form (often called somewhat optimistically an informed consent form), which includes some information about the contemplated treatment, probably evolved from simple consent forms more or less contemporaneously with the early court cases requiring disclosure, such as *Salgo* and *Natanson* (3,4; see Chapter 3). A major impetus to the development of consent forms came from the federal government's efforts to regulate recruitment practices in the research it sponsors. (See Chapter 11.)

There is no common-law requirement that consent forms be used. A number of courts have specifically stated that they are not necessary (5,6), and a number of opinions in informed consent cases have largely discounted their value. In the absence of any statutory provision governing the effect of a consent form signed by a patient, it has been held that the consent form "is simply one additional piece of evidence for the jury to consider.... [U]nless a person has been adequately apprised of the material risks and therapeutic alternatives incident to a proposed treatment, any consent given, be it oral or written, is necessarily ineffectual" (7).

Nonetheless, physicians and health-care facilities, probably on the advice of legal counsel, often insist upon the use of consent forms. Furthermore, eleven states (Florida, Idaho, Iowa, Louisiana, Maine, Nevada, North Carolina, Ohio, Texas, Utah, and Washington) have statutes that appear to encourage consent forms by according those that comply with the statutory requirements a "presumption of validity" (8). None, however, actually require that consent be obtained in writing (9).

Although these statutes were specifically enacted to protect physicians from lawsuits, their meaning and effect are ambiguous at best. Some statutes create from the existence of a signed consent form a so-called conclusive presumption of consent, while others refer to a presumption of valid consent or a presumption of informed consent. The implications of all these statutes are unclear in ways that should not be reassuring to a physician who wishes to rely on them. Furthermore, at least one statute creating a conclusive presumption has been determined to be unconstitutional because there was no rational relationship between the fact proved (that a consent form was signed) and the fact presumed (that the patient was adequately informed), and also because the statute denied patients a fair right of rebuttal (10).

The precise kind of presumption a statute creates could be extremely important to the litigants in an informed consent case. Because of the ambiguity of meaning arising from such terms as presumption of validity, presumption of valid consent, and presumption of informed consent, the consequences of a signed consent form could range from decisive to irrelevant. It would seem that a consent form creating a conclusive presumption that the patient both was adequately informed and gave consent could put a stop to a lawsuit almost immediately, since ordinarily if a presumption is conclusive, no evidence will be considered to the contrary.

Most of these statutes have not been construed in this manner by the courts. Rather, the statutes have been held to create a presumption of consent, but not to speak to the adequacy of disclosure. When physician-defendants attempt to halt informed consent cases by alleging that patients have signed consent forms in compliance with a statute, they are still required to establish that they in fact provided patients with information adequate to comply with the prevailing standard of care. If they can do so, then it is presumed or conclusively presumed that the patients consented to the procedure from the fact that they signed the consent form. This result may actually work to physicians' disadvantage, for it is usually not consent that is an issue, but the adequacy of disclosure. As a result of attempting to prove consent using the statutory presumption flowing from the signed consent form, the physician now must carry the burden of proving the adequacy of disclosure, a matter on which the patient would otherwise have had the burden of proof (11–14).

Because a signed consent form is intended to be conclusive merely as to the issue of consent and not the adequacy of disclosure, the form serves as a defense only to a charge of unauthorized treatment (i.e., battery) and not to a claim of inadequate disclosure (i.e., negligence). Conversely, a statute that is viewed only as creating a presumption of adequate disclosure, as some have been, is irrelevant in cases in which plaintiffs claim not that they were inadequately informed, but that they had not consented (15).

Under some of the statutes, evidence is admissible that fraud was involved in obtaining informed consent. For example, the Florida statute, which contains conclusive presumption language, states, "[the] presumption may be rebutted if there was a fraudulent misrepresentation of a material fact in obtaining the signature" (16). Thus, a patient who signs a form consenting to a sterilization may still testify that she was orally informed by her physician that there was no chance of getting pregnant again, even if the form itself notes that the procedure is not always effective (12). A patient told by his physician that no risks will accrue if the physician performs a recommended operation may testify to that effect and is entitled to have the jury instructed that the presumption of informed consent is overcome by such fraudulent disclosure (17). In such instances, the statute is essentially without effect. The plaintiff-patient must still bear the burden of producing evidence that he or she was not adequately informed—according to whatever standard of disclosure prevails in the jurisdiction—and juries must be able to find that this was the case more probably than not. The essential point is that the plaintiff is still entitled to get the claim of inadequate disclosure before a jury, an occurrence the presumption clauses in the statutes were probably intended to prevent.

Most statutes create not a conclusive presumption but merely a rebuttable presumption. Some of these statutes purportedly create a presumption of informed consent rather than mere consent. However, before the presumption may arise that the patient has been adequately informed, it is required that the form set forth the information the physician is obliged to provide the patient (18). Thus, at most, the consent form assists the defendant-physician by establishing a *prima facie* case of adequate disclosure and consent, which, however, may be overcome by the patient's evidence of fraud, misrepresentation, duress, or mistake. Fraud and misrepresentation involve deliberate action by the physician in misleading the patient. Pressure on the patient to sign the form may constitute duress. Even if there is no misrepresentation by the doctor, if the patient is under the mistaken apprehension that, for example, the form must be signed without any change, the presumption of validity might be overcome. Moreover, if the contents of the form are incomplete or ambiguous—for example, if it states only that the patient has been "adequately" informed—testimony must be taken to establish what the disclosure entailed, in this case to establish what "adequately" means.

Finally, and most importantly, a statute that creates a *prima facie* presumption of adequate disclosure and of consent works no change in existing law. It has always been the plaintiff-patient's responsibility to plead and prove inadequate disclosure and lack of consent (see Chapter 6), regardless of any statutorily created presumptions to that effect. The failure to present proof on these issues should lead to a dismissal of the case and the granting of a judgment in favor of the defendant-physician. Thus, there is no apparent benefit from the existence of many statutes.

In summary, then, a signed consent form's main legal use is as evidence that the patient at least had an opportunity to read the information on it. This is the case in most of the jurisdictions having statutes and the vast majority of jurisdictions without them. If the information presented in the consent form contains a description of the risk that actually came to pass and other information adequate for a reasonable person to make a decision, it will probably be helpful to a physician in the defense of a lawsuit. The plaintiff would only be able to attack the manner in which disclosure was made, or would have to establish that he or she was not given an opportunity to read the form or was misinformed about the nature of the document that was signed (19).

On the other hand, if the form presents inadequate or overly complex information, this evidence may support the plaintiff's case. If the form merely acknowledges that disclosure was made but fails to contain the content of what should have been disclosed, it is unlikely to provide the physician with any added advantage with respect to the main issue of litigation: what was disclosed and whether it was adequate (20). Often a consent form of any sort merely provides the opposing lawyer with a good target to attack. Consent forms may provide a false sense of security to physicians and hospital administrators, leading them to believe that a signed consent form constitutes informed consent. Vaccarino has concisely summarized the dangers of consent forms.

> By failing to distinguish between informed consent and its documentation, the legal profession has precipitated the most egregious misconception by physicians concerning informed consent, namely that if a consent form is signed, informed consent has been obtained. At the outset, the consent form must be recognized for what it is: nothing more than evidence that informed consent has been obtained (21, p. 862).

9.2 An Adjunctive Approach to the Use of Consent Forms

Given the rather limited role of consent forms in protecting practitioners from liability, and in light of the tendency of consent forms to turn the decisionmaking process into the less desirable decisionmaking event, some thought needs to be given to whether and how they should be used in medical settings.

One approach might be to eschew the use of consent forms altogether (11). Entering notes in patients' charts at the time consent is obtained may offer as much legal protection as a consent form, without the clinical complications that consent forms may entail. Clinicians can be encouraged to formulate a core disclosure for a particular treatment or procedures—items likely to be of importance to all patients for whom the treatment or procedure is recommended. This core disclosure can be modified by deleting some items or adding others, as the mutual monitoring process occurs (described in Chapter 8). The physician's note, written just after the disclosure, can simply record that the core disclosure took place, with any modifications noted. Since disclosure is likely to be an ongoing process, follow-up notes can record patients' later questions and the responses or additional information provided.

As attractive as this approach might be, in certain circumstances it is not feasible. As noted earlier, many facilities and research projects require the use of consent forms. And some clinicians may want to take advantage of whatever legal protection consent forms afford. Thus, a reasonable approach to their use must be formulated.

We believe that the consent form, when used at all, should be seen as an "adjunct" to oral disclosure and the doctor-patient conversation that should occur during all phases of their relationship. That is, physicians should convey all important information orally and not rely on consent forms to fill the gaps. Consent forms can be provided in advance of oral disclosure to prepare the patient for the process, or afterwards to aid reflection, integration, and the formulation of questions. In either event, consent forms should play an exclusively adjunctive role.

If the consent form is being used *after* disclosure, the physician— after discussing the nature, purpose, risks, benefits, and alternatives, and making a recommendation for a particular treatment— might say something like, "I use this form to remind myself and my patients that I am trying to provide the treatment that they want. This form is a written version of what I think we have agreed on as the appropriate treatment. Read it and tell me if that is what we have agreed on. If it isn't, then we need to do some more talking, because I haven't understood what you want."

Alternatively, some physicians may prefer to provide patients with consent forms *before* the major part of the disclosure, to enable them to pose questions and study the material on their own. Some research has suggested that overall patient comprehension can be improved with the use of this technique (22). Patients who receive consent forms prior to the formal stage of decision making can review them with friends, relatives, or other trusted caregivers, who may help them understand the information and better appreciate the consequences of a decision. Used in either of these ways, consent forms serve both as adjuncts to patient education and symbols of the agreement reached between physician and patient.

It has been suggested that the educative function of consent forms can be increased by the use of a two-part form (2). The first part consists of the ordinary written disclosure. The second part is a simple questionnaire designed to test patients' comprehension of the essential features of the situation. Although good evidence of its effectiveness is lacking, the concept of the two-part consent form reflects the importance of monitoring patient understanding (23). Nonetheless, it is mechanical and depersonalizing in nature. It could embarrass patients who may feel they are being tested and it could miss those obstacles to understanding that are not included on the prepared form. The monitoring of understanding, which is crucial to our concept of a meaningful decisionmaking process, might better be carried out in a discussion between doctor and patient. At the same time, physicians' roles in this discussion might be more effective if they were to begin with some ideas about areas of likely misunderstanding, and a thought process similar to that involved in constructing the two-part form could stimulate such awareness on their part.

9.3 Practical Issues

Three sets of issues related to the use of consent forms in the adjunctive manner proposed above need to be considered. These involve how the forms are constructed, the nuances involved in presenting them to patients, and the psychology of signing.

Construction of Consent Forms

When consent forms are used primarily for liability protection, there is a tendency to include large amounts of information, often of a technical nature, and to cover most conceivable risks. Evidence exists that patient understanding of information on consent forms is inversely related to their length (24). Overly inclusive consent forms may have the paradoxical effect of decreasing the level of patient understanding, perhaps even increasing the chance that a patient will feel misled, aggrieved, and inclined to sue. The way out of this dilemma is unclear. One runs the risk, in condensing, of deleting just that information that might in retrospect be alleged to have been crucial to the patient's decision. Forms may be too short as well as too long.

The "adjunctive" approach to consent forms (see Section 9.2) does relieve some of the tension about what to include. Since the form is seen as only an adjunct to doctor-patient discussion rather than a substitute for it, not everything of note need be included on the form. The statements on the form can emphasize that patients are being asked to make a choice about treatment and that information is being presented to aid them in the decisionmaking process. The form can then explain the nature of the procedure and detail the major risks and benefits, along with possible alternatives, while acknowledging that everything of interest to a particular patient may not be covered. A statement might be included, for example, that notes, "These are the major risks of (or alternatives to) this treatment. There are other problems that occur less frequently or are less severe. If you would like to know about them, your doctor will be happy to discuss them with you." Oregon, in fact, has adopted a statute that encourages this way of using consent forms—and oral disclosure, too (25).

Another option is to employ consent forms that allow the insertion of individualized information in blank spaces. Unfortunately, this method encourages clinicians to include an amount of information more appropriate to the size of the blank than the needs of the patient. An interesting attempt at constructing such a form has been published and may prove useful to physicians who desire to try this approach (26).

A related issue is the problem of complex language on consent forms. It is clearly more precise to write, "Research has shown that there is a statistically significant chance of a reduction in the circumference of a malignant sarcoma with this treatment," than to say, "The treatment is likely to improve your condition but not do away with your cancer altogether." Most physicians, accustomed to writing for professional audiences, automatically gravitate toward polysyllabic words, which make for greater precision. There is no doubt, however, that most patients would understand the second formulation better than the first.

Several studies have shown that the typical consent form is written with a complexity requiring at least college level, and often postgraduate, reading skills (1, 27). More careful attention to language might ameliorate this problem. Although there is no foolproof way of determining the readability of a consent form, the readability scales used by most educational researchers may be useful. The two best known are the Fry Readability Scale, which counts the number of words per sentence, and the Flesch Formula, which counts the number of syllables per 100 words (28, 29).

Grundner has studied samples of consent forms and suggests that a good one should not have fewer than 4.5 sentences per 100 words, not more than 150 syllables per 100 words (27). Such formulas are not infallible. For example, Levine has pointed out that at his institution consent forms generally say, "In the preparation of this consent form it was necessary to use several technical words; please ask for an explanation of any you do not understand" (30). On the Fry Scale, this scores in the upper college reading level, and it measures in the scholarly range using the Flesch Formula. One could substantially improve both readability scores by instead stating, "Some arcane words are on this page. I will construe them as you wish." But this version is probably even less likely to be understood.

A peculiar irony arises in the simplification of language on consent forms. Given that polysyllabic medical (or legal) jargon is often a shorthand for longer descriptions using simpler words, efforts to reduce the complexity of consent forms almost inevitably increase their length. For example, to simplify the sentence, "We are conducting an investigation of the pathogenesis and pathophysiology of hyperlipidemia," which consists of 12 words, one might have to resort to the following: "We are trying to find out more about persons who have unusually high levels of fats in their blood. In particular, we are studying what leads to the development of this condition and related changes in the way the body works." Although eminently clearer, the more colloquial version takes 40 words, more than three times the number in the original sentence. Since greater length decreases both overall comprehension and the likelihood that patients will read the entire consent form, some compromise between simplicity and length must be struck, and continued selectivity is needed about what should be included.

Some of these problems can be avoided by creating consent forms that are not forms at all. Clinicians and investigators have experimented with using video or audio tapes to supplement oral disclosure (31,32). Given that a large segment of the population has difficulty reading at even a high school level (33) and many patients may have impaired eyesight, there may be real advantages to these techniques. They may also have some value for proving in court that informed consent was obtained.

Presenting Consent Forms to Patients

How consent forms are presented to patients and by whom are matters of some concern. If the patient's signature is being recorded merely as a legal formality, it probably matters little who is present or precisely what is said. If consent forms are to be integrated into the decisionmaking process, these matters may assume larger meaning.

The way forms are presented relates to the overall attitudes of physicians and patients to both the forms and the informed consent process. The forms have an effect of their own in this regard. Even among clinicians with some overall commitment to the idea of informed consent, the temptation is strong to use the forms, once they are present, as a time-saving device—to thrust them into patients' hands, allowing a few minutes for looking them over, and then asking if there are any questions. Among busy physicians, this temptation may subvert the clinical instinct, leading them to substitute the signing of a form for a meaningful decisionmaking process. Thus, clinicians use expressions such as, "I got the informed consent," or "I got the patient to consent," as though consent were an object or mechanical process.

In a variety of ways physicians, nurses, and others may convey the impression that consent forms, even informed consent itself, are extraneous to the treatment process. Consent forms are frequently introduced with the phrase, "I have to ask you to sign this," or "We are required to tell you" (34, pp. 93–94). Consent forms and consent itself are seen as a bureaucratic process imposed on both physician and patient from the outside and completely unrelated to medical decision making and care. Patients quickly pick up such physician attitudes. In one study a patient, asked to describe the content of a series of forms he had signed when entering the hospital five minutes earlier, told the interviewer, "The paperwork has to be done, I guess, but I can't remember what was in it." Another patient signed the same set of documents even though she did not have her glasses and could not read without them. It was observed in this study that more than 50 percent of patients made no effort to read certain types of consent forms (34, pp. 91–94).

The adjunctive approach that we suggest to the use of consent forms might be thought likely to vitiate these problems, and if applied correctly, probably will. (See Section 9.2). But it is important to keep in mind the seductive tendency of consent forms to tear even well-meaning clinicians away from interactive decision making and toward a sterile version of consent, focused on the wording of a form, or worse, on the event of signing it.

The question of who obtains the patient's signature on the consent form raises complicated issues. It is common practice in many facilities for a nurse or someone other than the treating physician actually to obtain the patient's signature. If legal protection is all that is at stake, this may be acceptable, as long as there is some provision for responding to the patient's questions. If the consent form is to be integrated into physician-patient decision making, it is obviously desirable for the physician to be involved in the process. It can be argued, with some justification, that patients might be less intimidated about asking questions of a nonphysician, but that person may be less able to answer questions appropriately. Further, to the extent that physicians fail to learn patients' concerns by participating in the decisionmaking process, they will be unable to accommodate them in future disclosures, or situations in which they may have to make decisions on patients' behalf (e.g., when patients waive informed consent, or in emergencies). (Special considerations relating to this issue in the research setting are addressed in Chapter 12.)

The Psychological Meaning of Consent Forms

A patient's signature on a consent form does not constitute a legally binding commitment to go through with the treatment described. Patients are always free to withdraw their consent. Forms for consent to research often state this explicitly, but it is true whether contained on the form or not. Nonetheless, whatever the legal implications, psychologically a signed consent form represents a commitment on the part of the patient. Most people have learned in childhood that signing a document commits them to what is on the paper. One study has shown that the major factor inhibiting subject participation in survey research was the requirement that they sign consent forms (35).

The commitment symbolized by signing a form may have both positive and negative effects on patients' participation in medical decision making. Signing the form may encourage patients to reflect seriously on the proposed treatment before consenting. Patients who are deeply ambivalent about treatment may have an opportunity actively to resolve that ambivalence in the act of signing the form. To the extent that reflection and commitment to treatment are desirable ends, the use of consent forms may help reach them.

On the other hand, signing the form is often taken by patients to mean that their role in decision making is over. This idea fits their experience with other signed contracts. In buying a house or a car, the signature on the dotted line completes the transaction. Buyer and seller are both committed. There is usually no turning back, and therefore little incentive to continue to mull over the benefits and risks of the situation. In fact, the understandable human tendency is to persuade oneself that the best decision has been made and to put the issue out of one's mind.

A similar effect can be seen in medical treatment and research. Patients often see the signed form as binding them to go through with the treatment to which they have consented. There is a tendency to see the signing of the form as a time to relinquish one's concerns about medical treatment rather than as one phase of a continuing process of education about treatment and one decision amidst a series.

Two approaches might alleviate this tendency. First, of course, one could abandon the use of consent forms. For the reasons discussed previously, this may not always be either possible or desirable. Second, physicians could make extra efforts to insure that patients understand that the physician expects their continuous participation in decisions, and that they are not signing their bodies over to the medical system. If information continues to be provided, practitioners continue to inquire about patients' desires, and patients' efforts to participate are not dismissed out of hand, many patients may come to see the act of signing a consent form in its proper light.

References

1. Cassileth BR, Zupkin RV, Sutton-Smith K, et al.: Informed consent—why are its goals imperfectly realized? *N Engl J Med* 302:896–900, 1980.

2. Miller R, Wilner HS: The two-part consent form: a suggestion for promoting free and informed consent. *N Engl J Med* 290:964–966, 1974.

3. Salgo v. Leland Stanford Jr. University Board of Trustees, 317 P.2d 170 (1957).

4. Natanson v. Kline, 350 P.2d 1093 (1960).

5. Hernandez v. United States, 465 F. Supp. 1971 (D. Kan. 1979).

6. Maercklein v. Smith, 266 P.2d 1095 (Colo. 1954).

7. Sard v. Hardy, 379 A.2d 1014 (Md. App. 1977).

8. Meisel A, Kabnick LD: Informed consent to medical treatment: an analysis of recent legislation. *University of Pittsburgh Law Review* 41:407–564, 1980.

9. Doss v. Hartford Fire Insurance Co., 448 So. 2d 813 (La. App. 1984).

10. Cunningham v. Parikh, 472 So. 2d 748 (Fla. App. 1985).

11. Meisel A: More on making consent forms more readable. *IRB* 4(1):9, 1982.

12. Valcin v. Public Health Trust of Dade County, 473 So. 2d 1297 (Fla. Ct. App. 1984).

13. Estrada v. Jacques, 321 S.E.2d 240 (N.C. App. 1984).

14. LaCaze v. Collier, 416 So. 2d 619 (La. App. 1982), aff'd, 434 So. 2d 1039 (La. 1983).

15. Meretsky v. Ellenby, 370 So. 2d 1222 (Fla. App. 1979).

16. Fla. Stat. Ann. § 768.46 (4)(a) (West Cum. Supp. 1979).

17. Morganstine v. Rosomoff, 407 So.2d 941 (Fla. App. 1979).

18. Petty v. United States, 740 F.2d 1428 (8th Cir. 1984) (Iowa law).

19. Dandashi v. Fine, 397 So. 2d 442 (Fla. App. 1981).

20. Rhodes v. Doctors Hospital North, 18 O.O.3d 391 (Ohio App. 1980).

21. Vaccarino JM: Malpractice: the problem in perspective. *JAMA* 238:861–863, 1977.

22. Morrow G, Gootnick J, Schmale A: A simple technique for increasing cancer patients' knowledge of informed consent to treatment. *Cancer* 42:793–799, 1978.

23. Stuart RB: Protection of the right to informed consent to participate in research. *Behavior Ther* 9:73–82, 1978.

24. Epstein LC, Lasagna L: Obtaining informed consent—form or substance? *Arch Intern Med* 123:682–688, 1969.

25. Oregon Revised Statutes § 677.097 (1977).

26. Janik CJ, Swaney JH, Bond SJ, et al.: Informed consent: reality or illusion? *Information Design Journal* 2:197–207, 1981.

27. Grundner TM: On the readability of surgical consent forms. *N Engl J Med* 302:900–902, 1980.

28. Fry EA: A readability formula that saves time. *Journal of Reading* 11:513–516, 1968.

29. Flesch R: A new readability yardstick. *J Appl Psychol* 32:221–233, 1948.

30. Levine RJ: Research involving children: an interpretation of the new regulations. *IRB* 5(4):1–5, 1983.

31. Reynolds PM, Sanson-Fisher RW, Poole AD, et al.: Cancer and communication: information-giving in an oncology clinic. *Brit Med J* 282:1449–1451, 1981.

32. Malone ML: Informed consent and hospital consent forms: paper chasing in a video world. *Journal of Urban Law* 61:105–125, 1983.

33. Weiner MF, Lovett R: An examination of patients' understanding of information from health care providers. *Hosp Community Psychiatry* 35:619–620, 1984.

34. Lidz CW, Meisel A, Zerubavel E, et al.: *Informed Consent: A Study of Decisionmaking in Psychiatry.* New York, Guilford Press, 1984.

35. Singer E: Informed consent: consequences for response rate and response quality in social surveys. *American Sociological Review* 43:144–162, 1978.

10

Patients Who Refuse Treatment

From its inception, the law of informed consent has been based on two premises: first, that a patient has the right to receive sufficient information to make an informed choice about the treatment recommended; and second, that the patient may choose to accept or to decline the physician's recommendation. The legitimacy of this second premise should be underscored because it is too often belied by the everyday jargon of medical practice. *Getting a consent* is jargon that implies that patient agreement is the only acceptable outcome. Indeed, the term informed consent itself suggests that patients are expected to agree to be treated rather than to decline treatment. Unless patients are viewed as having the right to say no, as well as yes, and even yes with conditions, much of the rationale for informed consent evaporates.

This intuitively and logically obvious point is often overlooked in medical practice and judicial decisions. In medical practice, the right to refuse treatment often is ignored because it is inconsistent with the history and ethos of the medical profession (1; 2, pp. 1–29). The courts have recognized the relationship between the informed consent doctrine and the right to refuse treatment—that is, that the right not to be treated without consent is the same as the right not to be treated at all. However, they have been slow to enforce it.

10.1 Legal Attitudes Toward Refusal of Treatment

Although the right to refuse treatment is implicit in the legal doctrine of informed consent, because of the way informed consent cases reach the courts, judicial opinions rarely have the opportunity to acknowledge this right explicitly. A partial exception is a small number of so-called informed refusal cases, in which patients have declined treatment, to their detriment, and later contended that they would not have refused had adequate information been provided (3,4). Physicians can be held liable for inadequate disclosure in these cases. Their resolution has been based on the characterization of the right of refusal as a right whose exercise must be voluntary and informed.

The right to refuse treatment is addressed more directly in cases concerning patients' attempts to refuse care. The key determinant in these cases has been whether the refusing patient was terminally ill—that is, whether the patient would be likely to die in the near future even if the proposed intervention were undertaken. Courts have been remarkably unwilling to accept the right of nonterminally ill patients to refuse potentially life-saving care. On the other hand, patients whose death seems inevitable in the near future are frequently granted that right.

The series of cases involving terminally ill patients began with the landmark *Quinlan* decision of the New Jersey Supreme Court in 1976 (5). Since then, the courts of more than a dozen states have expressly held that incurably ill patients have a right to refuse treatment, and if incompetent, their surrogate has a right to decline further treatment on their behalf. No appellate court confronted with such a right-to-die case has refused to recognize the right, and in only one appellate case has a court failed to honor a patient's or surrogate's refusal (6). Often the courts have grounded their reasoning on the common-law right of patients to refuse treatment under the informed consent doctrine (7).

Nonterminally ill patients refusing potentially life-saving treatment have created more difficult situations for the courts. Many have involved the refusal of blood transfusions by Jehovah's Witnesses (8). A fair number have involved patients who needed to have gangrenous limbs amputated (9–13). Some involved parents refusing treatment of their children, often (but not always) motivated by religious belief (14,15).

In some of these cases, the courts determined that the patient was not competent, hence the physician could rely on neither the patient's consent nor refusal. Rather a guardian would have to be appointed to make a decision for the patient—usually a decision to treat. In the cases involving parental refusal of treatment of a minor child, the courts have usually, but not always, compelled treatment, because the treatment was considered either clearly life-saving or the only reasonable possibility for saving life, and the parents were deemed not to have the right to deprive the child of that opportunity. The cases in which courts have been more accepting of parental refusals have usually involved conditions that were not life-threatening for the child (16,17), but this too is not always the case (18).

The rest of the refusal cases have involved competent, adult patients. Despite Justice Cardozo's dictum that "Every human being of adult years and sound mind has a right to determine what shall be done with his body" (19), the courts have often compelled treatment of nonterminally ill, refusing adults. Sometimes they have grounded their decisions on the fact that the adults had dependent children (20,21). Occasionally they have resorted to intuiting what patients really wanted as opposed to what they said they wanted, especially in the case of religiously motivated refusals (22). Judging from both reported cases and news accounts of unreported cases, the courts have only rarely permitted nonterminally ill patients to decline what is intended to be life-saving treatment.

These cases diverge from the expectation that the courts would enforce the right of refusal as a corollary of the rights to disclosure and consent. The cause in part is that the factual settings of the informed consent cases differ from those in which an attempt is being made to compel treatment. The doctrine of informed consent has been developed by courts entirely in a retrospective fashion. In these cases the events have already occurred, and the patient has been harmed. The compelled treatment cases have addressed similar issues, but prospectively. A patient has refused treatment and a court must decide whether to uphold or override the refusal. Since hospitals ordinarily do not seek a court order to compel treatment unless the patient's life is in imminent jeopardy, there is an added urgency not present in most informed consent cases.

In the informed consent cases, judges have been psychologically freer (in the statutes, the same has been true of legislators) to indulge the wish to permit patients to decide freely about treatment. The events are all in the past, the patient has been injured, the past cannot be undone, and patient choice is honored. In contrast, in compelled treatment cases there is an opportunity to shape the future. The patient may be injured if permitted to refuse treatment, the decision lies in judicial hands, and patient choice gives way to the perceived greater good of saving a life.

In addition, the retrospective evaluation of informed consent cases allows courts to indulge the belief that the values of health and autonomy can both be served. That is, patient autonomy can be respected in a manner that will improve the doctor-patient relationship and ultimately lead to improved health care. The prospective focus of the compelled treatment cases forces the courts to choose between clearly defined options of autonomy and health, and perhaps understandably they have usually opted for the latter. In these cases the courts often pay homage to the principle of self-determination undergirding the right to refuse treatment. They then acknowledge that this right, as most others, is not absolute; there are a number of categories of exceptional situations in which other societal interests must eclipse individual autonomy. Almost invariably, the facts of the case are construed to fit one of these exceptions. Thus, the courts manage to honor the right but in the breach rather than the observance.

An independent line of cases—dealing with the right of involuntarily committed psychiatric patients to refuse treatment—addresses a situation that lies intermediate between the informed consent and the compelled treatment cases. The psychiatric patients in these cases are not terminally ill, which might incline the courts toward overriding their refusals. But neither is the proposed treatment, most commonly the use of antipsychotic medications, life-saving (even if restorative of sanity), which might lead the courts to uphold their decisions. The life-and-death imperatives driving the courts in the other cases are missing here. Despite the historic practice of treating committed patients without obtaining consent, almost all courts considering the issue have concluded that a right to refuse treatment exists (23–29). Although some courts have established a constitutional basis for the right, it is clearly drawn from the common-law right of disclosure and consent.

The courts, interestingly, have differed somewhat in their analysis of how this right should be enforced. Two lines of court decisions exist in this area. In the first, the right of refusal has been rooted in the basic assumptions of the law of informed consent, and efforts to treat involuntarily have been made to turn on an adjudication of incompetency (e.g., 23). In the second, token acknowledgment has been made of the right of refusal, but involuntary commitment has been seen as abrogating that right, so that involuntary treatment can be provided after a review of the appropriateness of the proposed regimen, irrespective of patient competency (e.g., 30). The latter view clearly supports the right of refusal less than the former.

Overall, then, the courts have manifested some ambivalence about the right to refuse treatment. Rather than enforcing it unquestioningly, they have tended to balance it against patients' interest in health (particularly in life), often abandoning the right to refuse when life might thereby be endangered. Some courts, however, have followed the implications of the legal doctrine of informed consent to their logical conclusions, accepting patients' rights to refuse treatment, even if their lives might thereby be lost.

10.2 The Dilemma of Refusal of Treatment in the Clinical Setting

If the courts have been caught between the values of autonomy and health, it should come as no surprise that the medical profession has been even more torn by the dilemma of patient refusal. Physicians are ordinarily deeply invested in promoting patients' health and convinced of the benefits of their interventions. There is an inherent frustration for physicians when patients reject treatment that physicians believe is badly needed. In fact, it is in just such situations that the conflict between autonomy and health appears most stark and unresolvable.

Respecting patients' refusals may involve a compromise of the interest in health, but this will not always be the case. Patients will often be choosing between treatments of limited or uncertain efficacy, often on the basis of the side effects that must be endured. A patient who suffers nausea or constipation from medication designed to reduce the pain of arthritis might well choose to forego it, if the effects of the drug are more troubling than the illness itself. Similarly, patients choosing among breast cancer treatments that are more or less disfiguring can be understood, given continuing controversy over the relative benefits of each approach, if they choose one that preserves their body intact. Whether or not the trade-off between treatments—or between the choice of treatment and no treatment—is roughly equivalent in medical terms, however, our society has given competent patients the right to make that choice.

Assessing Refusal of Treatment

Physicians can fulfill their obligation to protect health by assuring that again, as when patients choose to accept treatment, the patient's refusal is an informed one and made in accord with the patient's basic values. To accomplish this physicians must assess the bases for patients' refusals, and shape appropriate responses. This reaction to refusal can be viewed as an extension of the process model of informed consent. The mutual monitoring process need not end simply because the patient has turned down a recommendation for treatment.

As self-evident as the need to ascertain the bases for refusal may appear, studies of physicians' responses to patients' refusals suggest that targeted responses are the exception rather than the rule. Clinicians frequently react in an undifferentiated fashion to patients' refusals. Appelbaum and Roth have reported that physicians often attempted to persuade refusing patients to undergo the recommended treatments without first taking the time to ascertain the basis for the patients' refusals (31). This approach reduced physicians to general exhortations to their patients to accept treatment because of its importance to their care, or attempts to address the concerns the physicians thought were on patients' minds rather than those that were really at issue.

The reasons many physicians fail to pursue a more targeted approach to patient refusal are similar to those that generally inhibit doctor-patient communication. Doctors are busy and may seek to resolve an unexpected difficulty in the decision process in what seems like the most expeditious way possible. They may also believe that patients are unlikely to understand detailed explanations and that as a rule exhortation is more appropriate than education. And refusal of a physician's recommendations is often taken by the physician as a personal affront (32). Refusal of treatment is seen by physicians as a rejection of an offer of help, which in turn may be seen as a rejection of the person making the offer, particularly when physicians have made extra efforts on a patient's behalf. As a result physicians may feel angry, frustrated, and unwilling to explore the underlying basis of refusal.

Any effort to respond meaningfully to patients' refusals must overcome these tendencies and begin with a thorough exploration of the reasons for refusal (31,33,34). The sensitive mutual monitoring envisioned by the process model of informed consent can continue—as the refusal provides a focus for the interaction. Rather than emphasizing disclosure, the process now focuses on clarification of how the situation is seen by the patient. Patients are sometimes initially reluctant to reveal their reasons for refusal, feeling embarrassed about having inconvenienced their physicians or fearful of some sort of retaliation if their reasons are not good enough. Sometimes patients may even lack a conscious awareness of all the reasons. Physicians need to take the lead in identifying the bases for refusal.

In doing so, physicians ideally should be guided by a knowledge of the factors that tend to interfere with the expression of a knowledgeable, autonomous choice. The literature on refusal of treatment by medical patients, unfortunately, is heavily weighted with anecdotal papers (33–38). Systematic studies of the issue are rare (31). A larger number of studies have addressed the problem of treatment refusal by psychiatric patients, but they are not completely transferable to the general medical context (39–51). Nonetheless, existing knowledge does offer a starting point for the exploration of patients' refusals.

Research suggests that a number of factors interact to lead patients to make uninformed refusals. Studies indicate that the primary cause of poorly informed decision making is the common failure of physicians to inform patients about treatments or diagnostic procedures, much less to discuss purpose, benefits, and risks (31,52). Other studies have shown that physicians consistently underestimate the amount of information patients would like to have before making medical decisions (53,54). Patients can also be supplied with too much or too complex information, so that their ability to assimilate it is overwhelmed. They may receive conflicting information from one or several sources and end up bewildered about the facts surrounding their care (31,33). Physicians may have difficulty in conveying, and patients in understanding, the uncertainty inherent in medical procedures (2, pp. 165–206; 55). The empirical approach to treatment—involving trial-and-error approaches to selecting treatment—may be discomforting for both physicians and patients to talk about.

Some of the difficulties in communication may relate to structural factors within the health-care system. The organization of care in a modern medical center, for example, may require patients to be involved with a large number of physicians and other health-care workers. Confusion may arise over who really is the person to talk with about one's care, or conflicting information may be provided, or no information may be provided, if everyone assumes that someone else is taking the responsibility (56, p.103). Economic pressures may limit the amount of time physicians feel they can spend with patients either in the hospital or the office.

Clearly, a multiplicity of factors can contribute to a poorly informed decision by patients. Physicians can address their problems by monitoring patients' understanding, then shaping redisclosure to focus on these areas of confusion. To pinpoint issues requiring attention, physicians might ask patients, for example, to explain the nature and purpose of the proposed treatment. The extent of patients' knowledge can be further clarified by questioning them about their views of the possible consequences of treatment and of refusal. Besides uncovering simple misunderstandings, such questions may bring to the surface implicit beliefs about health, illness, and therapy that may lead patients to discount the information they are given (57,58). For example, a patient may believe that surgery on what the physician considers to be a potentially curable cancerous lesion is of no use because the diagnosis of cancer is equivalent to a death sentence that physicians are powerless to change.

Another concern about patient refusal is that it may fail to reflect patients' underlying values. Patients' emotional needs and styles of coping with them, the stresses of the treatment situation, and, in extreme cases, overt psychopathology can all result in decisions that are nonautonomous, in the sense that they do not reflect patients' value systems (59). Character traits such as rigidity, suspiciousness, ambivalance, a need to be in control (or conversely, passivity) can lead patients to refuse treatment even if, in the abstract, it is something they would desire (31). The maladaptiveness of these traits, which we all share to some degree, is heightened by the stress of hospitalization with its subtle depersonalization of patients and the threat to life and bodily integrity inherent in serious medical illness. The prospect of surgery, in particular, can produce severe anxiety, as patients confront fears of death, loss of control under anesthesia, and the prospect of unalterable change in their bodies (34).

Actual psychiatric illness, including psychosis, depression, and acute or chronic brain impairment, can exacerbate all of these reactions, leading to a decisionmaking process so compromised as to be considered incompetent. It should be emphasized, however, that refusal is only rarely a manifestation of psychiatric illness, and that psychiatric illness in itself is not sufficient to render patients incompetent. (See Chapter 5)

The frequency with which these threats to autonomous decision making arise requires physicians to assess additional aspects of patient refusals. Physicians can inquire about the way in which patients decided to reject the recommended care. Patients can be asked directly about the factors that entered into their decisions. To persuade them to speak frankly about their decisionmaking processes, physicians must convey the belief that reasonable patients may actually make decisions that conflict with their physicians' recommendations. Physicians may find it useful to consult with other caregivers, especially nurses, and with family members to uncover limitations on autonomous choice that may not be immediately apparent. Questioning of family members, for example, may reveal that the patient has undergone subtle psychological changes or is unrealistically depressed about the prospect of being a burden to the family.

Responding to Refusal

With the information acquired by assessing patients' reasons for refusal and the influences on them, physicians are in a position to formulate appropriate responses.

The initial response will often be simply to accept patients' decisions. If patients are well informed about the treatment options and have made choices that appear entirely consistent with their underlying values, they clearly have the right to refuse treatment. Many physicians will have no difficulty accepting patients' decisions in such circumstances. Nonetheless, if the patients' values involved differ from the physicians' values, some physicians may feel uncomfortable merely acquiescing in the decision.

Patients' values are of course deserving of respect, but it would seem excessive to demand that physicians make no attempt to persuade patients simply because a matter of values is at stake. Physicians ought to be seen as advocates for the value of health, and their efforts to persuade patients of the importance of receiving treatment encouraged. Although some common-sense stopping point is required at which physicians should acknowledge the disparity in underlying values and respect patients' choices, persuasion is a legitimate tool in the practice of medicine and should not be abandoned. Advocacy, however, must not be permitted to turn into coercion. Unfortunately, the line between persuasion and coercion is exceedingly fine, and physicians must be extremely sensitive to overstepping it. Threats to withhold all future care if the patient continues to refuse a recommended treatment are inappropriate.

The effort to persuade the patient is not a one-way process. Patients may be able to alter physicians' perceptions of the best course of treatment, and physicians need to remain open to this possibility. Best of all, the two participants may be able to reach a compromise that satisfies all interests. A medication the patient initially refused, for example, may be started at a lower dose than the physician proposed, with further increments dependent on the absence of side effects.

Sometimes, in contrast to this situation, it will be clear that patients are making uninformed decisions. At this point physicians must reinitiate the effort to educate the patient. A good assessment will have revealed the basis for the patient's lack of understanding and will suggest appropriate corrective measures. Additional information might be provided, the explanation simplified, or other people, such as family members, called in to aid the patient's understanding. All previous suggestions about offering information and monitoring patients' understanding are relevant here. (See Chapter 8.)

It will sometimes also be apparent that, patients are well informed but their decisions are not reflective of their own values. For example, to the extent that maladaptive character traits have led patients to become angry with their caregivers and thus reject attention, or that overt psychopathological factors are implicated, consultation with a psychiatrist may be of use. Evidence indicates that such consultations are underutilized in these circumstances, with psychiatrists being called in only when patients are clearly psychotic; their expertise in diagnosing and managing depression and problematic character traits tends to be ignored (31).

Once the problem has been identified, a response can be devised. Alteration of the environment may help. A patient in one study who described herself as a "night owl" consistently refused to have blood drawn when awakened early in the morning, which was the hospital's routine, but agreed to undergo the procedure when it was arranged for the technician to come later in the day (31). Family members may be enlisted to ease patients' anxieties, making it easier for them then to act according to their underlying values. A brief psychotherapeutic intervention may have the same effect. The use of neuroleptic medication or the cessation of a medication that is clouding the patient's sensorium may restore decisionmaking capacity. The list of potential responses to impairments either in understanding or in autonomous action can be added to ad infinitum without encompassing all possibilities. The key lies in the individualization of response, which in turn depends on a careful assessment of patients' decision making.

What should physicians' responses be when all efforts at persuasion, education, and removal of obstacles to the expression of underlying values fail? If patients are believed to be incompetent, of course, a substitute decision can be sought either judicially or extrajudicially. (See Chapter 5.) Physicians should beware too rapid a resort to the legal process. It can lessen the chances of resolving the situation short of an extended and expensive court proceeding, which can tear apart the fabric of the doctor-patient relationship, and is an unquestionable assault on patient autonomy. The law is a last resort to be reserved for otherwise intractable cases (e.g., when efforts to restore patient competency have failed) with potentially serious outcomes.

Assuming the patient is competent, the clinician is faced with two other options: continuing to treat in accord with the patient's wishes (or a negotiated compromise) without utilizing the rejected treatment, or discharging the patient from further care. The latter option should be employed only when the physician is convinced that the refused treatment is absolutely crucial to the patient's care and that there are no alternatives the physician could ethically pursue. These occasions will be rare. When they occur, reasonable efforts must be made to find a physician willing to accept the stated limitations, so that the patient will not be abandoned. Careful self-scrutiny ought to take place before a decision to terminate care, to be sure that the choice is based on the absence of other reasonable options and not on the physician's desire to strike back at a frustrating patient.

Conclusion

Patients' refusals are among the most difficult situations physicians must handle. They must come to grips with the limits on their authority to order interventions and on their power singlehandedly to combat disease and restore health. Even physicians who are generally supportive of the idea of informed consent may balk at its implications when patients refuse care physicians believe will be highly beneficial. The reality, however, is that no human being is omnipotent. We all must face real limitations on our power to pursue our goals and advance our values. Having done what they can to insure informed decision making by patients who are refusing treatment, as outlined above, physicians can do no more. Their moral and legal obligations have been fulfilled. If in consequence patients are not treated precisely the way their physicians would have desired, that is the price we pay as a society for supporting individual freedom of choice.

10.3 Informed Consent and Refusal of Treatment

Patients' refusal of treatment is the nub of many physicians' opposition to the idea of informed consent. (See Chapter 7.) Not particularly resistant to sharing information with patients, these physicians are concerned that the emphasis on patients' choice inherent in the doctrine encourages refusals of treatment. Given their orientation toward the value of health, this outcome seems to them undesirable. In medical terms, it could be considered a side effect of the idea of informed consent.

Theoretically it should be possible to study the effect of the idea of informed consent on the frequency of patient refusals, but it has not been done. Clinicians have from time to time published anecdotal accounts of patients who have been led to refuse treatment as a result of the information provided them; the cases reported are usually those with adverse outcomes (60–62). Certainly, both the ethical and legal doctrines at the root of the legal requirement of informed consent anticipate that some patients will refuse treatment after receiving appropriate information (one might say that the opportunity to refuse is the point of the whole thing). It cannot be denied that some patients who otherwise would have accepted care might refuse apparently desirable treatment after participating in the process of informing and seeking consent.

On the other hand, and most noteworthy, the empirical and anecdotal studies of patients who refuse treatment almost never portray the process of obtaining informed consent as playing a causative role. The opposite appears to be true. Refusal of treatment has repeatedly been linked to patients' being inadequately, not overly, informed. In other words, it is *failure* to live up to the idea of informed consent that has been shown to precipitate refusal of treatment. Physicians who neglect the careful discussion of treatment options, including their nature, purpose, risks, and benefits, seem much more likely to have patients refuse their recommendations for care than their colleagues who adhere more closely to the idea of informed consent.

Of course, merely providing adequate information does not insure that patients will accept treatment or that their decisions will be reasonable. As noted above, refusal that is ill informed or in conflict with patients' underlying values is usually complex. A patient's fears of surgery and pressure from family members who distrust physicians may combine with information that leaves the patient confused about the purpose of the procedure, and a patient who at heart really does desire to be treated may refuse. Although each factor by itself might not have led to refusal, taken as a group they do. (The prevention of poorly informed or nonautonomous refusal does not require that all the precipitating factors be dealt with. Removal of one may be sufficient to help the patient to make a better informed and more genuine choice.) Of all the problems likely to be involved in these cases, the provision of information is the one most under physicians' control and thus easiest for them to remedy. If the dilemmas raised by ill-informed, nonautonomous refusal are to be addressed anywhere, the process must begin here.

Informed consent does indeed have a relation to refusal of treatment, but not the expected one. Rather than acting most commonly as a stimulus to refusing treatment, informed consent—particularly in the process model (see Chapter 8)—may actually serve a preventive function. Our present knowledge suggests that well-informed patients are less likely to refuse treatment than those who are poorly informed. Patients for whom the process of mutual monitoring has been successful—whose physicians are aware of their beliefs, values, and attitudes toward treatment, and who in turn are cognizant of their physicians' beliefs, values, and attitudes—will rarely get to the point of using refusal as a weapon. If they do not wish to follow their physicians' recommendations and cannot negotiate an alternative, they may reject the treatment offered, but usually this will be done in the context of an ongoing physician-patient relationship. These facts should serve to reassure clinicians who may have tended to see informed consent as an alien construct imposed on them by the law and working to the detriment of patient care, rather than a natural extension of the sensitive clinician's desire to build a working relationship with his or her patients.

References

1. Appelbaum PS, Roth LH: Involuntary treatment in medicine and psychiatry. *Am J Psychiatry* 141:202–205, 1984.

2. Katz J: *The Silent World of Doctor and Patient.* New York, Free Press, 1984.

3. Truman v. Thomas, 611 P.2d 902 (Cal. 1980).

4. Crisher v. Spak, 471 N.Y.S.2d 741 (Sup. Ct. 1983).

5. Matter of Quinlan, 355 A.2d 647 (N.J. 1976).

6. Matter of Storar, 420 N.E.2d 64 (N.Y. 1981).

7. E.g., Matter of Conroy, 486 A.2d 1209 (N.J. 1985).

8. Power of courts or other public agencies, in the absence of statutory authority, to order compulsory medical care for adult. *American Law Reports 3d* 9:1391–1398, 1966.

9. In re Quackenbush, 383 A.2d 785, 788 (N.J. Super. 1978).

10. State Department of Human Services v. Northern, 563 S.W.2d 197 (Tenn. App. 1978).

11. In re Nemser, 273 N.Y.S.2d 624 (N.Y. Sup. Ct. 1966).

12. Lane v. Candura, 376 N.E.2d 1232 (Mass. App. 1978).

13. Matter of Schiller, 372 A.2d 360 (N.J. Super. 1977).

14. Power of court or other public agency to order medical treatment over parental religious objections for child whose life is not immediately endangered. *American Law Reports 3d* 52:1118–1124, 1973.

15. Power of court or other public agency to order medical treatment for child over parental objections not based on religious grounds. *American Law Reports 3d* 97:421–426, 1980.

16. In re Green, 292 A.2d 387 (Pa. 1972).

17. Matter of Seiferth, 127 N.E.2d 820 (N.Y. 1955).

18. Matter of Sampson, 317 N.Y.S.2d 641 (Family Ct. 1970).

19. Schloendorff v. Society of New York Hospital, 105 N.E. 92, 93 (N.Y. 1914).

20. E.g., In re President & Directors of Georgetown College, Inc., 331 F.2d 1000 (D.C. Cir. 1964).

21. E.g., Raleigh Fitkin-Paul Morgan Memorial Hospital v. Anderson, 201 A.2d 537 (N.J. 1964).

22. E.g., United States v. George, 239 F. Supp. 752 (D. Conn. 1965).

23. Rogers v. Okin, 478 F. Supp. 1342 (D. Mass. 1979), *aff'd in part and rev'd in part,* 634 F.2d 650 (1st Cir. 1980), *vacated and remanded,* 457 U.S. 291 (1982), *opinion on certification sub nom.* Rogers v. Commissioner of the Department of Mental Health, 458 N.E.2d 308 (Mass. 1983), and *on remand* Rogers v. Okin, 738 F.2d 1 (1st Cir. 1984).

24. Rennie v. Klein, 462 F. Supp. 1131 (D.N.J. 1978), *later proceeding*, 476 F. Supp. 1294 (D.N.J. 1979), *modified and remanded*, 653 F.2d 836 (3d Cir. 1981), *vacated*, 458 U.S. 1119 (1982), *on remand*, 720 F.2d 266 (3d Cir. 1983).

25. Davis v. Hubbard, 506 F. Supp. 915 (N.D. Ohio 1980).

26. Colyar v. Third Judicial Dist. Court, 469 F. Supp. 424 (D. Utah, 1979).

27. A.E. and R.R. v. Mitchell, No. C-78-466 (D. Utah, June 12, 1979).

28. Jamison v. Farabee, No. C-78-0445-WHO (N.D. Cal., April 26, 1983) (consent decree).

29. In re K.K.B., 609 P.2d 747 (Okla. 1980).

30. Project Release v. Prevost, 722 F.2d 960 (2d Cir. 1983).

31. Appelbaum PS, Roth LH: Treatment refusal in medical hospitals, in President's Commission for the Study of Ethical Problems in Medicine and Biomedical and Behavioral Research, *Making Health Care Decisions: The Ethical and Legal Implications of Informed Consent in the Patient-Practitioner Relationship.* Vol. 2, *Appendices.* Washington, D.C., U.S. Government Printing Office, 1982; summarized in Appelbaum PS, Roth LH: Patients who refuse treatment in medical hospitals. *JAMA* 250:1296–1301, 1983.

32. Meister R: Psychiatrists' reactions to their patients' refusal of drugs. *Israel Annals of Psychiatry and Related Disciplines* 10:373–381, 1972.

33. Himmelhoch J, Davis N, Tucker G, et al.: Butting heads: patients who refuse necessary procedures. *Psychiatry Med* 1:241–249, 1970.

34. Scully JH: *Psychiatric Problems in Primary Practice, No. 3: Psychiatric Problems in Surgery* (pamphlet). Manati, Puerto Rico, Roche Products Inc., 1982.

35. McCartney JR: Refusal of treatment: suicide or competent choice? *Gen Hosp Psychiatry* 4:338–343, 1979.

36. Goldberg RJ: Systematic understanding of cancer patients who refuse treatment. *Psychother Psychosom* 39:180–189, 1983.

37. Lansky SB, Vats T, Cairns NV: Refusal of treatment: a new dilemma for oncologists. *Am J Pediatr Hemat/Oncol* 1:277–282, 1979.

38. Hershkowitz M: To die at home: rejection of medical intervention by geriatric patients who had serious organic disease. *J Am Geriatr Soc* 32:457–459, 1984.

39. Appelbaum PS, Hoge SK: Empirical research on the effects of legal policy on the right to refuse treatment, in Parry J (ed.), *The Right to Refuse Antipsychotic Medication.* Washington, D.C., American Bar Association, 1986.

40. Gill MJ: Side effects of a right to refuse treatment lawsuit: the Boston State Hospital experience, in Doudera AE, Swazey JP (eds.), *Refusing Treatment in Mental Health Institutions—Values in Conflict.* Ann Arbor, Association of University Programs in Health Administration Press, 1982.

41. Appelbaum PS, Gutheil TG: Drug refusal: a study of psychiatric in-patients. *Am J Psychiatry* 137:340–346, 1980.

42. Marder SR, Mebane A, Chien CP, et al.: A comparison of patients who refuse and consent to neuroleptic treatment. *Am J Psychiatry* 140:470–472, 1983.

43. Marder SR, Swann E, Winslade WJ, et al.: A study of medication refusal by involuntary psychiatric patients. *Hosp Community Psychiatry* 35:724–726, 1984.

44. Rodenhauser P: Treatment refusal in a forensic hospital: ill-use of the lasting right. *Bull Am Acad Psychiatry Law* 12:59–63, 1984.

45. Rodenhauser P, Schwenker CE, Khamis HJ: Drug treatment refusal and the course of forensic hospitalization: basic issues (unpublished manuscript).

46. Hassenfeld IN, Grumet B: A study of the right to refuse treatment. *Bull Am Acad Psychiatry Law* 12:65–74, 1984.

47. Keisling R: Characteristics and outcome of patients who refuse medication. *Hosp Community Psychiatry* 34:847–848, 1983.

48. Zito JM, Routt WW, Roerig JL: Clinical characteristics of psychotic patients who refuse antipsychotic drug therapy. *Am J Psychiatry* 142:822–826, 1985.

49. Zito JM, Lentz SL, Routt WW, et al.: The treatment review panel: a solution to treatment refusal? *Bull Am Acad Psychiatry Law* 12:349–358, 1984.

50. Hargreaves WA, Shumway M: The Jamison-Farabee consent decree: an attempt to protect the right of involuntary psychiatric patients to refuse antipsychotic medication. Presented at the Annual Meeting of the American Psychiatric Association, Dallas, Tex., May 1985.

51. Rodenhauser P, Heller A: Management of forensic psychiatry patients who refuse medication—two scenarios. *J Forensic Sci* 29:237–244, 1984.

52. Lidz CW, Meisel A: Informed consent and the structure of medical care, in President's Commission for the Study of Ethical Problems in Medicine and Biomedical and Behavioral Research, *Making Health Care Decisions: The Ethical and Legal Implications of Informed Consent in the Patient-Practitioner Relationship.* Vol. 2, *Appendices.* Washington, D.C., U.S. Government Printing Office, 1982.

53. Harris L, and associates: Views of informed consent and decisionmaking: parallel surveys of physicians and the public, in President's Commission for the Study of Ethical Problems in Medicine and Biomedical and Behavioral Research, *Making Health Care Decisions: The Ethical and Legal Implications of Informed Consent in the Patient-Practitioner Relationship.* Vol. 2, *Appendices.* Washington, D.C., U.S. Government Printing Office, 1982.

54. Strull WM, Lo B, Charles G: Do patients want to participate in medical decisionmaking? *JAMA* 252:2990–2994, 1984.

55. Bursztajn H, Feinbloom RI, Hamm RM, et al.: *Medical Choices, Medical Chances: How Patients, Families, and Physicians Can Cope with Uncertainty.* New York, Delacorte Press, 1981.

56. Lidz C, Meisel A, Zerubavel E, et al.: *Informed Consent: A Study of Decisionmaking in Psychiatry.* New York, Guilford, 1984.

57. Stimson GV: Obeying doctor's orders: a view from the other side. *Soc Sci Med* 8:97–104, 1974.

58. Becker MH (ed): *The Health Belief Model and Personal Health Behavior.* Thorofare, N.J., Charles B. Black, 1974.

59. Miller BL: Autonomy and the refusal of lifesaving treatment. *Hastings Center Report* 11(4):22–28, 1981.

60. Katz RL: Informed consent—is it bad medicine? *West J Med*, 126:426–428, 1977.

61. Patten BM, Stump W: Death related to informed consent. *Tex Med*, 74:49–50, 1978.

62. Kaplan SR, Greenwald RA, Rogers AJ: Neglected aspects of informed consent, *N Engl J Med* 296:1127, 1977.

IV

CONSENT TO RESEARCH

11

The Law

11.1 The Independent Evolution of Informed Consent to Research

Oddly enough, despite the apparent similarities in the issues raised, informed consent in the research setting has evolved quite separately from informed consent to treatment. Consent to treatment is largely a creature of case law, with some subsequent statutory modification. Consent to research has been shaped by professional codes, statutes, and administrative regulations, with the courts playing a less important role.

Systematic medical research, of course, is a newer phenomenon than medical treatment. The eighteenth century saw some of the first efforts—to demonstrate the etiology of diseases. One was Lind's controlled study of the effects of citrus juices in preventing scurvy (1). Pierre Louis' classic study, in the 1820s, of the efficacy of blood-letting as a treatment for pneumonia demonstrated the potential of clinical investigation, but his medical colleagues were slow to follow his lead (2). By the turn of the twentieth century, the pace of experimentation with human subjects was quickening.

The etiologies of beriberi and pellagra, for example, were discovered using human volunteers.

Prior to World War II, little attention was paid to the circumstances under which research should be carried out, including the issue of consent. There are a few statements extant from leading physicians of the time, such as Paul Ehrlich, endorsing the disclosure of information about the risks and benefits of experimental treatment. Public concern in Germany culminated in the promulgation in 1931 of guidelines that required clear explanations of innovative or experimental treatments (3). But the retrospective accounts of physician-investigators who were active at the time make clear that obtaining consent was simply not part of the everyday conduct of research (4).

This situation began to change with the trials of Nazi physicians at Nuremberg that began in 1946 and helped focus the attention of the world on the ethics of medical research. Testimony at the trials revealed that concentration camp inmates and prisoners of war had been used as subjects in so-called experiments, many of which were devoid of valid scientific purpose, without consent and with wanton cruelty. The procedures performed included the deliberate inoculation of inmates with typhus bacilli to propagate strains of the bacteria, the irradiation of gonads to devise rapid and inexpensive means of mass sterilization, and the exposure of inmates to cold water and low air pressure to observe the events that would lead to their deaths (5, pp. 1274–1288; 6). The military judges at Nuremberg, outraged by the revelation of these studies, which seemed to them to cross the line between experimentation and torture, asked their expert witnesses—most notably the American physicians Andrew Ivy and Leo Alexander—to articulate the universal standard of ethical research practices from which the Nazi experimenters had deviated.

Ivy obtained the endorsement of the American Medical Association for three basic principles of human experimentation: "(1) The voluntary consent of the person on whom the experiment is to be performed must be obtained; (2) The danger of each experiment must have been investigated previously by means of animal experimentation; and (3) The experiment must be performed under proper medical protection and management" (7). With considerable modification and elaboration by the judges of the Nuremberg tribunal, these standards were incorporated in the court's final judgment against the Nazi physicians, in the case known as *United States* v. *Karl Brandt* (8). These standards have come to be known as the Nuremberg Code.

Two of the ten sections of the code dealt with informed consent; the remaining eight sections established limits on the power of researchers to inflict harm on subjects in the name of science. The first section laid out a clear-cut requirement for obtaining informed consent:

> The voluntary consent of the human subject is absolutely essential. This means that the person involved should have legal capacity to give consent, should be so situated as to be able to exercise free power of choice without the intervention of any element of force, fraud, deceit, duress, overreaching, or other ulterior form of constraint or coercion and should have sufficient knowledge and comprehension of the elements of the subject matter involved as to make an understanding and enlightened decision. This latter element requires that before the acceptance of an affirmative decision by the experimental subject there should be made known to him the nature, duration, and purpose of the experiment; the method and means by which it is to be conducted; all inconveniences and hazards reasonably to be expected; and the effects upon his health or person which may possibly come from his participation in the experiment (9).

A subsequent provision mandated that the subject have the right to terminate participation "if he has reached the physical or mental state where continuation of the experiment seems to him to be impossible" (9).

"All agree," wrote the court, "that certain basic principles must be observed in order to satisfy moral, ethical, and legal concepts" (9). Ironically, it seems that the court, casting about for a principled basis on which to condemn intuitively repugnant behavior, mistook the aspirations of a few leaders of medicine with regard to disclosure and consent for the practices of the vast majority of researchers (1). In any event, even if viewed as a statement of an ideal, the Nuremberg Code had limited immediate impact on worldwide research practices. As a decision of a court whose jurisdiction arose *sui generis*, the code was not enforceable under the law of individual nations.

Some researchers were not satisfied with the provisions of the Nuremberg Code. Beecher, for example, pointed to the absolute requirement for informed consent as possibly precluding research with whole classes of people, such as the mentally ill. In addition, he objected (somewhat less cogently) to the requirement of an understanding and enlightened decision, since he believed that many research subjects were incapable of grasping the details of medical treatment and the techniques of clinical research sufficiently to meet that goal (11).

Dissatisfaction with the Nuremberg Code stimulated worldwide discussion about the ethics of conducting research and led to the promulgation of subsequent codes in a large number of countries (1,12). Most of these national codes echoed Nuremberg to some extent, but a number deviated significantly, toward greater leniency with regard to consent. The statement of the British Medical Research Council, for example, distinguished between experimentation that was likely to benefit the subject and experimentation that was not, and eliminated the requirement for informed consent in the former (13).

As national codes developed, the need for an international restatement of common principles became evident. In 1964 the World Medical Association adopted the Declaration of Helsinki, which serves as the definitive expression of international concerns (14). Like the British statement, the declaration distinguished between "clinical research combined with patient care" and "nontherapeutic clinical research," holding that in the former, "If at all possible, consistent with patient psychology, the doctor should obtain the patient's freely given consent after the patient has been given a full explanation" (14). The qualifying phrases leave considerable room for researchers to decide that they need not obtain consent in a particular case.

For nontherapeutic research, the declaration insisted, "The nature, purpose and the risk of clinical research must be explained to the subject by the doctor," and "Clinical research on a human being cannot be undertaken without his free consent after he has been fully informed" (14). Guardians were permitted to consent to either type of research for legally incompetent persons. The Declaration of Helsinki marked the culmination of the code-making process, the first stage of efforts to regulate the recruitment

and treatment of human research subjects. Paradoxically, by permitting consent to be foregone in "clinical research combined with
patient care," the declaration endorsed a standard that fell below
the historic common-law standard for consent to treatment. This
oddity highlights the distinct and often disparate development of
the regulation of consent to research.

Had cases of abuse in research made their way through the
courts, the rules governing treatment and research would probably
have been more similar. The pre–1964 case law is all but barren
of suits involving actual research settings. A small number of cases
from the nineteenth century on involved unique treatment approaches formulated by the defendants and directed at improving
a particular patient's situation, not at the systematic acquisition of
generalizable knowledge for the benefit of others (15). The decisions in many of these cases discouraged the idea of innovation,
holding physicians closely to prevailing standards of care, from
which they deviated at their own risk. A New York court in 1871,
for example, stated, "Any deviation from the established mode or
practice shall be deemed sufficient to charge the surgeon with
negligence, in case of an injury arising to the patient" (16). More
recent cases have been a bit more hospitable to innovation, but
required patient knowledge of and consent to the novel practice.
"We recognize the fact that, if the general practice of medicine
and surgery is to progress," wrote the Michigan Supreme Court
in 1935, "there must be a certain amount of experimentation carried on; but such experiments must be done with the knowledge
and consent of the patient or those responsible for him, and must
not vary too radically from the accepted method of procedure"
(17). Still, despite their language, this case and the cases that
followed it dealt with innovation and not with the conduct of systematic research.

In the early 1960s, the nonbinding codes were almost everywhere
the sole means of regulating research. As noted, their provisions
concerning informed consent varied substantially. The lasting impact of the codes was their setting the stage for the extensive
statutory and administrative regulation that was to ensue.

The United States took the lead in the development of administrative regulations. Their antecedents date to the opening of the
Clinical Center of the National Institutes of Health (NIH) in 1953,

when loose guidelines were formulated for subject consent (18). Since it was believed that experimental procedures used with patients should not be subject to regulation, lest the doctor-patient relationship be impaired, the application of the guidelines was limited to volunteers without physical illnesses. Even for this group, written consent was required only when there was a possibility of an unusual hazard (19). Research funded by NIH but conducted by researchers elsewhere in the country remained free of regulation, with "researchers to be guided by their own professional judgment and controlled by their own ethical standards as well as those of their institution" (20, p. 409).

The amount of extramural research funded by the NIH grew, and it awarded a contract in 1960 for a study of ad hoc procedures for the regulation of research in major medical centers around the country. Fifty-two departments of medicine responded to a questionnaire. Only nine had procedural documents to guide their investigators in the ethical design and implementation of research protocols. Five others said they were planning to develop guidelines or favored doing so. Only two of the existing documents covered all clinical research being performed in the institution. Twenty-two departments had committees that reviewed the protocols being implemented in their institutions, but none became involved in questions concerning the recruitment of subjects. (20, pp. 406–408).

In 1962, the same year the survey was performed, a congressional committee was conducting hearings to review the regulatory procedures of the Food and Drug Administration (FDA), the agency responsible for monitoring the testing of new medications in the United States. The hearings were already under way when the news broke of a large number of congenital deformities caused in Europe by the drug Thalidomide. In response to public concerns generated by the Thalidomide tragedy, Congress enacted the Drug Amendments of 1962 (20, pp. 410–412). The new law tightened controls on the approval process for new medications in the United States. It also required, in clinical trials of new drugs, that subjects be informed of the investigative purpose for which the medications were being used, and their consent obtained (21). A large loophole was created by permitting researchers to dispense with consent "where they deem it not feasible or, in their professional judgment, contrary to the best interest of such human beings." Although an FDA official indicated that the agency intended to interpret the exceptions in the statute narrowly, the FDA itself did not tighten its regulations until 1966, when it elaborated on the consent requirement, drawing heavily on language in the Nuremberg and Helsinki Codes (20, 21).

Meanwhile, the NIH had formed an internal study group to devise a uniform policy on the regulation of experimentation. In 1966 the Public Health Service, parent body of the NIH, issued a brief statement of policy on both intramural and extramural research programs funded by the NIH (18). Grant recipients were required to

> provide prior review of the judgment of the principal investigator or program director by a committee of his institutional associates. This review should assure an independent determination: (1) of the rights and welfare of the individual or individuals involved, (2) of the appropriateness of the methods used to secure informed consent, and (3) of the risks and potential medical benefits of the investigation (18, p. 52).

With this step, the federal government cast the mold for all subsequent regulation of the research process. From this point on, regulation provided for a decentralized, institution-based, prospective review of research, with informed consent explicitly required as part of the process of subject recruitment. The Public Health Service regulations, extended to encompass all research funded by the Department of Health, Education, and Welfare, were modified on several occasions, with required procedures growing steadily more complex. The last major revision was undertaken in 1981. At that point most of the discrepancies were resolved between FDA regulation of clinical trials of new medications and NIH regulation of biomedical research. From the original brief statement of policy in 1966, in 1981 the revisions had grown to seven pages of small print in the *Federal Register*, with 20 pages of accompanying explanations (26).

Much of the pressure to expand the regulations came from continuing revelations about unethical research practices. In 1963, it was revealed that investigators at the Jewish Chronic Disease Hospital in Brooklyn had injected live cancer cells into elderly patients without their knowledge or consent (22, pp. 9–66). Henry Beecher, a distinguished researcher and anesthesiologist at Harvard Medical School, published in 1966 an enumeration of research practices of questionable character culled from papers printed in major American medical journals (23). His work suggested that the consciousness-raising effect of the national codes had not been sufficient to stop such practices as the use of highly dangerous, unproven, nontherapeutic investigative techniques without the consent of experimental subjects. In 1971, it was revealed that in six southern states black men with syphilitic infections had been observed by their physician-investigators for nearly four decades and had been left untreated, even after effective and safe treatment for syphilis became available, in order to observe the natural history of the disease (24). The U.S. Army acknowledged in 1975 that unwitting civilians had been given hallucinogenic compounds to observe their psychological reactions. At least one of the subjects had died (25).

It is little wonder that the regulations have been expanded to specify the details of review of experimental protocols, including the composition of the review committees, the scope of their responsibilities, the criteria to be considered prior to approval of research protocols, the records to be kept, and the manner in which informed consent is to be obtained from subjects (26). There continues to be little litigation about research practices, probably due in part to the adoption of federal regulations and their salutary effect. (This is not to say that the informing of prospective research subjects is always conducted in compliance with the spirit of the informed consent doctrine.)

Whatever the reasons, only about a half dozen reported legal cases have arisen from the conduct of medical research in the last few decades (27–33). Most of them involve the use of innovative procedures outside of a clinical trial. None involve research that was subjected to an institutional review board (IRB) review. Thus, they serve merely as a reminder that judicial regulation of biomedical research continues to play only the most minor role, in comparison with IRB review. Nonetheless, the courts remain available to provide recourse to research subjects who have been harmed by inadequate disclosure—of potential research risks, therapeutic options (if any), and the possible lack of any benefits from research participation—or inappropriate pressure to participate.

11.2 Current Regulation

The most important conceptual difference between the regulation of consent in research and treatment settings is that consent to research is reviewed prospectively, while consent to treatment is ordinarily subject only to retrospective review, if any.

These differing approaches, of course, are a reflection of the origins of regulation in these areas. The very fact that consent to treatment has been left to judicial control, while consent to research is regulated by administrative bodies, points to the fundamental distinctions between the treatment and research processes. In the treatment setting, physician, patient, and society share a general consensus about the overall goal, promoting the patient's health, and conflicts that arise usually turn on the question of whether that goal was pursued in the most appropriate way. Patients may charge, for example, that physicians undertook their task of diagnosis and treatment negligently, or that in their therapeutic zeal they failed sufficiently to respect patient autonomy. By granting patients access to the courts for independent review of their care, society provides a means of compensating patients who have suffered harms resulting from negligent practices, and not incidentally of deterring physicians from engaging in them. The general confluence of patients' and physicians' goals and the relative rarity of conflicts lend themselves to a system with minimal oversight and selective retrospective review.

In the research setting things are somewhat different. Researcher and subject may share some goals—for example, the advancement of knowledge—but are likely to be in conflict about others. Subjects of clinical research (in which treatment is provided) will naturally be concerned about receiving optimal care for their conditions. Their physicians must balance their desire to treat optimally with the need to maintain a valid experimental situation (34, pp. 50–56; 35). Subjects of nonclinical research (in which no treatment is provided) will have a natural interest in avoiding harm. Although researchers will generally share that goal, they may be somewhat more inclined than subjects to take risks in order to generate desired data.

The conflicts between researchers' interests and those of their subjects have been firmly in the public mind since Nuremberg. It has been the horror stories of researchers failing to resolve those conflicts to their subjects' benefit that have given continued impetus to regulation. The perception of real conflicts of interest in the research setting, therefore, has stimulated more rigorous review than is found in the treatment setting. Prospective oversight of all research has evolved primarily to prevent exploitation of research subjects.

There are obvious advantages and disadvantages to the prospective approach. As noted, prospective review can be effective in preventing harms, without excluding the possibility of compensation should harm occur. Such review also provides control over researchers who might not alter undesirable practices merely because of the remote possibility of a lawsuit for damages. Furthermore, prospective review permits the rapid formulation of a body of coherent rules, while retrospective review is limited to consideration of the particular circumstances presented by the case at hand.

Universal prospective review does have substantial costs, including the cost of the personnel required to carry out the review and the value of time lost awaiting approval. Another possible cost is that the complacent assumption may be engendered, in both reviewers and reviewed, that the goals, design, and methods of conducting the research and obtaining informed consent from prospective subjects are unimpeachably in accord with ethical principles. There is a growing body of literature suggesting that in the review process IRBs focus primarily on the content of consent forms and pay inadequate attention to numerous other aspects of research that affect its overall conformance with ethical norms (36, 37).

The prospective review process in the United States has been created primarily by federal regulation, although some states have supplemented it with statutes of their own. Since biomedical research is funded primarily by the U.S. Department of Health and Human Services (DHHS), the rules promulgated by that agency have proven to be the most influential. Technically, DHHS regulations apply only to research undertaken with DHHS support. Two factors have combined to extend the influence of the DHHS rules. First, the agency requires institutions applying for funding to provide assurance that even research not funded through DHHS will be given some prospective review. Although different standards could be applied to these protocols, it has proven easier for institutions simply to adopt a uniform standard. Second, even institutions not required to submit assurances, when casting about for standards of their own, are likely to adopt the DHHS model because of its official imprimatur. It should be noted that several states have rules that may come into play for research outside the scope of DHHS regulation (38, pp. 503–577). The FDA has a discrete set of regulations, for the most part similar to the DHHS rules, but with occasional differences (see below).

There may be a large number of institutions in which biomedical research occurs that are not subject to the federal regulatory scheme. The volume of this research is probably not particularly great. There are no data available on what measures, if any, they have voluntarily adopted for the protection of human subjects. Even in institutions subject to the federal regulations, the possibility exists for covert research—research which the investigator does not submit for review by the IRB and which does not otherwise come to its attention.

Institutional Review Boards

With the promulgation of the initial DHHS (then DHEW) guidelines in 1966, a decision was made to decentralize the review process. Institutions receiving federal funds were required to establish IRBs to undertake research review. The most recent revision of the regulations, issued in 1981, requires that IRBs have "at least five members, with varying backgrounds to promote complete and adequate review of research activities commonly conducted by the institution" (26). The members must reflect diversity of professional and cultural backgrounds, sex, and race. At least some members must be knowledgeable about applicable law and regulations, as well as the relevant standards of professional conduct and practice. At least one member must have primary concerns that are nonscientific, and at least one must be otherwise unaffiliated with the institution. If the IRB regularly reviews research proposals involving "a vulnerable category of subjects," one member must be primarily concerned with the welfare of those subjects (26).

The role of the IRB is to review research proposals to insure that they conform with the federal regulations. Several substantive criteria must be addresssed. Researchers' protocols must minimize risk to subjects; any existing risks must be reasonable in relation to anticipated benefits; selection of subjects must be equitable; informed consent must be sought and appropriately documented; and, where appropriate, special provisions must be made for monitoring the privacy and safety of subjects, and protecting so-called vulnerable subjects (see Section 11.3) from undue coercion. The secretary of DHHS has the authority to waive any requirements of the regulations in particular cases. Mechanisms for appeal of IRB decisions have been established by some institutions, but subsequent review and approval by the original IRB is required (39).

Exempt Research

Several limited categories of research are exempt from IRB review and from federal regulatory control in general. These include:

(1) research conducted in educational settings, involving normal educational practices;

(2) research involving the use of educational tests, as long as the subjects cannot be identified individually;

(3) research involving survey or interview procedures, if responses are not recorded in a way that would permit subsequent identification of the subjects; responses would not place the subject at risk of criminal or civil liability or damage to financial standing or employability; and the research does not deal with sensitive aspects of the subject's behavior;

(4) research involving observations of public behavior, with the same qualifications as in (3) above; and

(5) research involving the collection or study of existing data, documents, records, pathological specimens, and diagnostic specimens, as long as the information is publicly available or is recorded in such a way as to render the subjects unidentifiable (26 §101[b]).

These provisions were adopted in response to complaints that regulations devised for biomedical research were being inappropriately applied to behavioral and social science studies. Protests continue to be heard from social scientists that the current exemptions are not broad enough, forcing them to obtain consent in ways that impair their effectiveness and for studies that present no real risks to subjects (40). Although the federal regulations specify the exemptions listed above, it is the prerogative of the IRB to determine whether a particular project is exempt. The federal regulations do not prevent institutions or other bodies from regulating exempt research. This fact has further aroused the ire of the social science community.

Expedited Review

In addition to exemptions, DHHS regulations provide for expedited IRB review of other kinds of research projects. Such review may be conducted by the chairperson or another designated member of the committee without awaiting a scheduled IRB meeting. Current categories of research eligible for expedited review include projects in which no more than minimal risk is likely to accrue to subjects and the procedures involve only the following:

(1) collection of hair, nail clippings, or deciduous teeth;

(2) collection of excreta and external secretions;

(3) recording of data from subjects 18 years of age or older using noninvasive, routine clinical practices (e.g., electrocardiography), excluding x-ray procedures;

(4) collection of blood samples by venipuncture in reasonable amounts;

(5) collection of dental plaque and calculus;

(6) voice recordings;

(7) moderate exercise by healthy volunteers;

(8) the study of existing data or documents;

(9) research on individual or group characteristics or behavior, where no manipulation of behavior or stress for the subjects is involved;

(10) research on drugs or devices for which the FDA would not require special exemptions (41).

Expedited review does not relieve investigators of the responsibility of formulating appropriate methods for obtaining informed consent.

The Regulatory Approach to Disclosure

To aid IRBs in determining what constitutes informed consent, in both the ordinary and expedited review process, current regulations specify in detail what is to be disclosed and how. Prospective subjects must be given information related to the "eight basic elements of informed consent" set forth in the regulations:

(1) a statement that the study constitutes research, an explanation of its purposes and the expected duration of subject involvement, and a description of the procedures involved, with experimental procedures identified as such;

(2) a description of risks and discomforts that are "reasonably foreseeable";

(3) a description of possible benefits to subjects and others;

(4) disclosure of appropriate alternative treatments, if any;

(5) a statement describing the extent of confidentiality of records generated;

(6) an explanation of whether compensation or treatment will be available if injuries occur;

(7) a note as to who can be contacted with questions or reports of injuries; and

(8) a statement as to the voluntary nature of participation and the subject's right of withdrawal at any time (26, §116 [a]).

In addition, the regulations list six optional elements of information that may be included if appropriate:

(1) a statement that unforeseen risks may arise;

(2) a description of circumstances in which subjects' participation may be terminated without their consent;

(3) a note as to any additional costs to the subject as a result of participation;

(4) a description of the consequences of premature withdrawal;

(5) a statement that subjects will be informed of any findings that may affect their willingness to continue; and

(6) a notation of the number of subjects to be involved in the research (26, §116 [b]).

Consent Forms

The DHHS regulations focus primarily on what information must be given to subjects. Another focus is the manner in which information is given. This issue has two aspects. The first involves the format for providing information. In most cases a written consent form is required, setting forth the information relevant to the proposed research, and is to be signed by subjects if they are to participate. With IRB approval, oral disclosure and a short form may be used; the short form, signed by the subject, contains a statement that the required elements of disclosure have been made orally. Presumably this option for oral consent is a response to the objections of some investigators that for many studies in clinical settings, or social research projects involving naturalistic observation, subjects are not capable of assimilating or not likely to attend to a lengthy written document. In specified circumstances even the short form can be dispensed with—when the study presents no more than minimal risk, or when the signed document would be the only record linking the subject to the project and the major risk to the subject is breach of confidentiality. Waiver of the requirement for a signed consent form is solely at the discretion of the IRB.

Deception Research

A reading of the regulatory definition of informed consent might suggest that deception research, in which subjects are deliberately uninformed or misinformed about the nature of the study in order to measure their unsuspecting reactions to the experimental circumstances, is prohibited. In fact, IRBs often make use of the flexibility in the regulations to "approve a consent procedure which does not include, or which alters, some or all of the elements of informed consent" (26). Such adjustments are permitted when the research involves no more than minimal risk, subjects' rights and welfare will not be affected adversely, the research could not otherwise be performed, and whenever appropriate, subjects will be debriefed about the deception at the conclusion of the study. Data suggest that informed consent regulations have not inhibited the use of deception; to the contrary, deception research has increased markedly and steadily over the last four decades (42).

Voluntariness, Understanding, and Competency

The other way DHHS regulations affect the manner in which information is provided involves the problem of voluntariness. The regulations require that consent be sought "only under circumstances that provide the prospective subject or the [subject's legally authorized] representative sufficient opportunity to consider whether or not to participate and that minimize the possibility of coercion or undue influence" (26).

The regulations address the related problems of understanding and competency almost as cursorily as voluntariness. They merely require that information be provided in language that subjects are likely to understand. There is no requirement that either the investigator or the IRB undertake any effort to ascertain adequacy of understanding, and no guidance for action in the event that a subject's understanding is deficient.

The regulations are equally vague about the related issue of competency. They direct that when patients are incompetent, their legally authorized representative may consent on their behalf to participation as a research subject. Who is a legally authorized representative is a matter to be determined by reference to state rather than federal law. The method for determining who is an appropriate representative, or surrogate, is a matter of great confusion in many places. (See Chapter 5.) The problem is further complicated by the question of whether even judicially appointed guardians have the authority to consent to their wards' participation as research subjects, especially where procedures are not intended to benefit subjects. Finally, the regulations are silent on the question of whether or not patients may be entered into research protocols in an emergency when it is impossible to obtain either their consent—because of their severely impaired mental or physical condition—or the consent of a legally authorized representative, because the latter is not present and the need for medical care is urgent (43).

The informed consent requirements promulgated by the FDA, governing the use of investigational drugs and devices, are largely similar to the DHHS regulations (44). Because of the need for flexibility regarding the testing of potentially life-saving drugs and devices, the FDA permits use without informed consent when the drug or device is essential to preserve a subject's life and it would be infeasible to obtain informed consent. It is less clear whether this provision permits entry of such a patient into a randomized clinical trial without informed consent—as opposed to merely permitting the use of an experimental drug. The FDA also requires subjects to be informed that the FDA may review their medical records as part of its oversight function.

How Effective Is the Regulatory Approach?

The regulatory approach, embodied in both the DHHS and FDA rules, allows much more precise specification of controls on consent than does an approach that relies heavily on case law. One unfortunate aspect of the decentralized review system and the absence of an appellate body, however, has been the lack of a formal mechanism to distribute information among review boards and to establish precedent in the resolution of difficult cases (45). This lack has contributed to the perception that the responses obtained from IRBs vary from institution to institution, depending on the composition of the panel and other idiosyncratic factors (46,47). There has been some informal effort to share information about problematic cases (48).

The performance of IRBs with regard to informed consent has been explored by a number of researchers. There is substantial variation in the care with which IRBs address issues of informed consent (49). Empirical studies of IRB function and decisions have supported the impression that IRBs tend to concern themselves more with the wording of consent forms than more substantial issues of consent and the conduct of research (35,36). In addition, there is a consensus that IRBs rarely exercise their available powers to require monitoring of the manner in which patients are approached as potential subjects, are provided with relevant information before making their decisions to participate, have their questions about participation answered both before and after deciding, or are permitted to exercise their right to discontinue participation.

11.3 Special Populations

More detailed and exacting supplementary regulations have been issued by the DHHS for the protection of several categories of subjects thought to be more vulnerable to pressure, less able to comprehend, or potentially subject to greater harm from participation in research than members of the general population, even the general population of patients. These groups include pregnant women, fetuses, products of in vitro fertilization, children, and prisoners (50,51,52).

Special protections for mentally ill and mentally handicapped persons were the subject of extensive recommendations by the National Commission for the Protection of Human Subjects of Biomedical and Behavioral Research (53). None of those recommendations were implemented. This outcome was the result in large part of opposition from researchers on mental disorders, who claimed that the populations in question were no more vulnerable than most persons with severe medical disorders and that the suggested limitations would seriously restrict research on mental disorders (54). Mentally impaired subjects continue to be covered under the general regulations, which, in the case of incompetency, allow consent to be obtained from a subject's legally authorized representative, presumably a guardian or equivalent person with the power to consent on the subject's behalf under the laws of the jurisdiction.

The regulations permit IRBs to require investigators to take special precautions to protect subjects "likely to be vulnerable to coercion or undue influence" (26, §111[b]). The National Institutes of Health are testing a trial plan that provides for the use of durable powers of attorney—instruments that permit appointment of a surrogate—for subjects who can anticipate future incompetency (e.g., subjects with progressive dementia), or who may be competent to designate a surrogate but not to decide about participation themselves. This plan, if successful, will allow research to continue with these populations but permit patients' interests to be protected by decision makers of their choice (55). It should be noted that while the federal regulations do not establish different procedures for research with the mentally ill, many states regulate research performed in state facilities (e.g., 56).

Research involving fetuses, pregnant women, and products of human in vitro fertilization has been subject to both substantive and procedural regulation (50). Pregnant women (and thus their fetuses) cannot be involved in federally supported research unless the purpose of the project is to meet the health needs of the woman or her fetus, or the risk to the fetus is minimal. Consent is required from both the mother and father of the fetus, who must be legally competent. The father's consent may be waived if the health needs of the mother are at stake, he cannot be located, or the pregnancy was the result of rape. IRBs are given a special set of responsibilities when research involves fetuses, pregnant women, or in vitro fertilization. IRBs must determine that adequate attention has been given to the means of selecting subjects and that "adequate provision has been made by the applicant or offeror for monitoring the actual informed consent process"—as by engaging independent persons to oversee the consent process. Some states have also enacted laws restricting the conduct of fetal research, often motivated by concerns related to the regulation of abortion (38).

Research with children has been made the subject of additional federal regulation, with special provisions concerning informed consent (51). Previous practice, supported by common law, required parental consent alone for children's participation. Investigations of the competency of children to understand information about research suggest that their abilities may reach adult levels at about age 14—well before the age of legal majority in most states (57). Even younger children appear to be able to grasp many of the concepts related to decision making. This discovery has led to the belief that children above a certain age ought to have the right to participate in the decision, rather than leaving it entirely to their parents or legal guardians (58). Some questions exist, as well, about the presumed confluence of interests between children and parents. Parents cannot always be trusted to guard their children's rights or interests (59). Parents may often even be unaware that they have agreed to let their children participate in clinical investigations (60). As a result of these factors, federal regulations now permit IRBs to require the assent of the child-subject ("a child's affirmative agreement to participate in research") in addition to the consent of parent or guardian (51). In making the determination to require such assent, IRBs are to take into account "the ages, maturity, and psychological state of the children involved" (51). Objections to these regulations have been voiced on the basis that permitting children to make decisions independent of their parents is destructive of family integrity, but this appears to be a minority view (61). The regulations also restrict the performance of research that presents more than minimal risk to child-subjects.

The elderly have also been singled out for special attention. It has been alleged that differences in physical and psychological functioning contribute to susceptibility to coercion and the likelihood of consent without genuine understanding (62). It has been suggested that the elderly might be included in the category of vulnerable subjects specially protected in the DHHS regulations that refer to situations "[w]here some or all of the subjects are likely to be vulnerable to coercion or undue influence" (38, p. 563). Nonetheless, federal regulations make no special provisions for obtaining consent from the elderly. Local IRBs may choose to establish additional requirements in particular projects. Research projects involving large numbers of elderly persons who are likely to be incompetent (e.g., studies of moderate or advanced senile dementia) may be required to screen for subjects' competency prior to seeking consent and to make provisions for consent from an appropriate surrogate in the case of probable incompetency. Interestingly, efforts to provide special protection for the elderly have stirred up opposition on the grounds that they are based on inaccurate, stereotypic characterizations of elderly persons (62). Special protections, in this view, contribute to a myth that the elderly in general are not capable of making decisions for themselves and therefore need to be protected from themselves.

Concerns have also been raised about prisoners. Their competency has been questioned on the grounds that "judgment about an acceptable degree of risk requires contact with the free world as opposed to the prison environment. What may be perceived as an acceptable risk for a person inside prison may be totally unacceptable for that same person outside" (63). This view is supported by the opinion in the major legal case on this issue, which has received a great deal of notoriety. Faced with the question of whether to permit a prisoner to participate in an experimental psychosurgical procedure, a Michigan trial court, in the *Kaimowitz* case, stated, "Institutionalization tends to strip the individual of the support which permits him to maintain his sense of self-worth and the values of his own physical and mental integrity. An involuntarily confined mental patient [the subject was actually a prisoner in this case] has diminished capacity for making a decision about irreversible experimental psychosurgery" (64). Burt has argued further that the message given a prisoner about his or her self-worth distorts the ability to weigh the risks and benefits of participation in research (65). The ability of prisoners voluntarily to consent has also been brought into question. Rewards such as money, escape from boredom, and the goodwill of one's jailers have been claimed to constitute coercive pressures (63). The *Kaimowitz* court held that the prisoner is in "an inherently coercive atmosphere even though no direct pressures may be placed upon him" (64). Preliminary empirical research has suggested that prisoners are likely to consent to research for emotional rather than rational reasons and to ignore risk-benefit ratios in making their decision (66). It is unclear whether these characteristics of prison populations distinguish them from the population at large.

The result of these concerns (which were shared by the National Commission for the Protection of Human Subjects of Biomedical and Behavioral Research [67]) was a severe restriction imposed in 1980 on the use of prisoners for research funded by DHHS or supervised by the FDA (52,68). Only limited classes of investigations were permitted. Studies of the possible causes of effects of incarceration and of prisons as institutional structures were permitted, if no more than minimal risk was involved. Studies of conditions affecting prisoners as a class and of practices that might improve their well-being and health could be conducted, but required the approval of the secretary of DHHS, or of the FDA, following consultation with experts.

Not all parties have agreed with the restrictions placed on prison research. A federal court, prior to the issuance of the new regulations, rejected the argument that prisoners could not provide valid consent (32). Inmates of the Jackson State Prison in Michigan, where much testing of new drugs had been performed, sued to prevent the implementation of the FDA's 1980 regulations (69). They alleged that they should have the right to decide whether the risks of participation outweigh the rewards, including improved living conditions and spending money. (Harm to subjects at Jackson was exceedingly rare.) In response, the FDA reformulated its regulations (which, however, have never been officially adopted) to permit some research not related to prison conditions when compelling reasons were present (70).

From a more theoretical perspective, the reasoning of those who would restrict prison research has been challenged on the grounds that it proves too much: Accepted on its face, the reasoning in *Kaimowitz*, for example, would disenfranchise prisoners from making almost any meaningful decision (71). Prisoners' competency, it is argued, is not different in its dimensions from that of nonprisoners. Moreover, an analysis of coercion should take into account the difference between unfair coercion and the inevitable coercion of circumstances, for example, the likelihood of certain benefits if a particular decision is made (71). These arguments have not altered the current regulatory climate, and prison-based research is for the most part no longer being carried out.

Conclusion

In the last two decades an extensive system of prospective regulation of research with human subjects has been erected. Much of the effort has been devoted to defining the proper nature of informed consent to research. Yet, as was true with informed consent in the clinical setting, the legal requirements provide only a part of the picture with which practitioners must be concerned. The existing regulations lay out the types of information that must be communicated to potential subjects. They give no guidance about the specific information that should be conveyed, the emphasis different elements of disclosure should receive, or the method of accomplishing a meaningful explanation. Selection of a proper approach depends on an understanding of the differences between consent to treatment and consent to research.

References

1. Bassiouni MC, Baffes TG, Evrard JT: An appraisal of human experimentation in international law and practice: the need for international regulation of human experimentation. *Journal of Criminal Law and Criminology* 72:1597–1666, 1981.
2. Louis PCA: *Researches on the Effects of Bloodletting in Some Inflammatory Diseases*. Boston, Hilliard, Gray, 1836.
3. Howard-Jones N: Human experimentation in historical and ethical perspectives. *Soc Sci Med* 16:1429–1448, 1982.
4. Parson W: Uninformed consent in 1942. *N Engl J Med* 310:1397, 1984.
5. Shirer WL: *The Rise and Fall of the Third Reich*. Greenwich, Conn., Fawcett Publications, 1960.
6. Ivy AC: Nazi war crimes of a medical nature. *Federation Bulletin* 33:133–146, 1947.
7. Judicial Council, American Medical Association: Requirements for experiments on human beings, in Ladimer I, Newman RW (eds.), *Clinical Investigation in Medicine: Legal, Ethical and Moral Aspects*. Boston, Boston University Law-Medicine Research Institute, 1963, p. 142.
8. United States v. Karl Brandt, et al., in U.S. Adjutant General's Department, *Trials of War Criminals Under Control Council Law No. 10 (October 1946–April 1949)*. Vol. 2, *The Medical Case*. Washington, D.C., U.S. Government Printing Office, 1947.
9. The Nuremberg Code, in Reiser SJ, Dyck AJ, Curran WJ (eds.), *Ethics in Medicine: Historical Perspectives and Contemporary Concerns*. Cambridge, Mass., M.I.T. Press, 1977, pp. 272–273.
10. Alexander L: Limitations of experimentation on human beings with special reference to psychiatric patients. *Dis Nerv Syst* 27(Suppl.):61–65, 1966.
11. Beecher HK: Some fallacies and errors in the application of the principle of consent in human experimentation. *Clin Pharmacol Ther* 3:141–145, 1962.
12. Frenkel DA: Human experimentation: codes of ethics. *Legal Medical Quarterly* 1:7–14, 1977.
13. British Medical Research Council: Memorandum on clinical investigations, in Ladimer I, Newman RW (eds.), *Clinical Investigation in Medicine: Legal, Ethical and Moral Aspects*. Boston, Boston University Law-Medicine Research Institute, 1963, pp. 152–154.
14. World Medical Association: Declaration of Helsinki: Recommendations guiding medical doctors in biomedical research involving human subjects, in Reiser SJ, Dyck AJ, Curran WJ (eds.), *Ethics in Medicine: Historical Perspectives and Contemporary Concerns*. Cambridge, Mass., M.I.T. Press, 1977, pp. 328–329.

15. Ladimer I: Ethical and legal aspects of medical research on human beings, in Ladimer I, Newman RW (eds.), *Clinical Investigation in Medicine: Legal, Ethical and Moral Aspects*. Boston, Boston University Law-Medicine Research Institute, 1963, pp. 179–209.

16. Carpenter v. Blake, 60 Barb. 488 (N.Y. 1871).

17. Fortner v. Koch, 272 Mich. 273, 261 N.W. 762 (1935).

18. Frankel MS: The development of policy guidelines governing human experimentation in the United States: A case study of public policy-making for science and technology. *Ethics in Science & Medicine* 2:43–59, 1975.

19. Sessoms SM: Guiding principles in medical research involving humans, National Institutes of Health, in Ladimer I, Newman RW (eds.), *Clinical Investigation in Medicine: Legal, Ethical and Moral Aspects*. Boston, Boston University Law-Medicine Research Institute, 1963, pp. 143–147.

20. Curran WJ: Governmental regulation of the use of human subjects in medical research: the approach of two federal agencies, in Freund PA (ed.), *Experimentation with Human Subjects*. New York, Braziller, 1970, pp. 402–454.

21. Kelsey FO: Patient consent provisions of the Federal Food, Drug, and Cosmetic Act, in Ladimer I, Newman RW (eds.): *Clinical Investigation in Medicine: Legal, Ethical and Moral Aspects*. Boston, Boston University Law-Medicine Research Institute, 1963, pp. 336–344.

22. Katz J: *Experimentation with Human Beings*. New York, Russell Sage Foundation, 1972.

23. Beecher HK: Ethics and clinical research. *N Engl J Med* 274:1354–1360, 1966.

24. Jones JH: *Bad Blood*. New York, Free Press, 1981.

25. Barrett v. Hoffman, 521 F. Supp. 307 (S.D.N.Y. 1981).

26. 45 Code of Federal Regulations §§ 46.101–46.409.

27. Halushka v. University of Saskatchewan, 52 W.W.R. 608 (Sask. 1965).

28. Karp v. Cooley, 349 F. Supp. 827 (S.D. Tex. 1972), *aff'd*, 493 F.2d 408 (5th Cir. 1974).

29. Valenti v. Prudden, 397 N.Y.S.2d 181 (App. Div. 1977).

30. Prisoner loses suit claiming coercion to participate in research. *IRB* 1(5):8, 1979.

31. Illinois lawsuits resolved by guidelines on research with mentally ill. *IRB* 1(6):8–9, 1979.

32. Bailey v. Lally, 481 F. Supp. 203 (D. Md. 1979).

33. Scott v. Casey, 562 F. Supp. 475 (N.D. Ga. 1983).

34. Fried C: *Medical Experimentation: Personal Integrity and Social Policy*. New York, American Elsevier, 1974.

35. Appelbaum PS, Roth LH, Lidz CW: The therapeutic misconception: informed consent in psychiatric research. *Int J Law Psychiatry* 5:319–329, 1982.

36. Gray BH, Cooke RA, Tannenbaum AS: Research involving human subjects. *Science* 201:1094–1101, 1978.

37. Appelbaum PS, Roth LH: The structure of informed consent in psychiatric research. *Behavioral Sciences and the Law* 1(4):9–19, 1983.

38. Rozovsky FA: *Consent to Treatment: A Practical Guide*. Boston, Little Brown, 1984.

39. Reatig N: Can investigators appeal adverse IRB decisions? *IRB* 2(3):8–9, 1980.

40. Patullo EL: Who risks what in social research? *Hastings Center Report* 10(2):15–19, 1980.

41. United States Department of Health and Human Services, Public Health Service: Activities which may be reviewed through expedited review procedures set forth in HHS regulations for protection of human research subjects. *Federal Register* 46:8392, January 26, 1981.

42. Adair JG, Dushenko TW, Lindsay RCL: Ethical regulations and their impact on research practice. *Am Psychologist* 40:59–72, 1985.

43. Abramson NS, Meisel A, Safar P: Deferred consent: a new approach for resuscitation research on comatose patients. *JAMA* 255:2466–2471, 1986.

44. 21 Code of Federal Regulations §§ 50.1–50.27, 56.101–56.124 (1984).

45. Calabresi G: Reflections on medical experimentation in humans, in Freund PA (ed.), *Experimentation with Human Subjects*. New York, Braziller, 1970, pp. 178–196.

46. Mathews D, Sorenson JR, Swazey JP: We shall overcome: multi-institutional review of a genetic counseling study. *IRB* 1(2):1–3, 12, 1979.

47. Goldman J, Katz MD: Inconsistency and institutional review boards. *JAMA* 248:197–202, 1982.

48. See discussions in *IRB: A Review of Human Subjects Research*, published by The Hastings Center, beginning March 1979.

49. President's Commission for the Study of Ethical Problems in Medicine and Biomedical and Behavioral Research: *Implementing Human Research Regulations: The Adequacy and Uniformity of Federal Rules and of their Implementation*. Washington, D.C., U.S. Government Printing Office, March 1983.

50. 45 Code of Federal Regulations §§ 46.201–46.211 (1984).

51. 45 Code of Federal Regulations §§ 46.401–46.407 (1984).

52. 45 Code of Federal Regulations §§ 46.301–46.306 (1984).

53. National Commission for the Protection of Human Subjects of Biomedical and Behavioral Research: *Report and Recommendations: Research Involving Those Institutionalized as Mentally Infirm*. DHEW Publication No. (OS) 78–0006. Washington, D.C., U.S. Government Printing Office, 1978.

54. Public response critical of HEW regulations on mentally disabled. *IRB* 1(2):8–9, 1979.

55. Fletcher JC, Dommel FW, Cowell DD: Consent to research with impaired human subjects. *IRB* 7(6):1–6, 1985.

56. 55 Pa. Code § 7100.113.3.

57. Melton GB, Koocher GP, Saks MJ: *Children's Competence to Consent*. New York, Plenum, 1983.

58. National Commission for the Protection of Human Subjects of Biomedical and Behavioral Research: *Research Involving Children: Report and Recommendations*. DHEW Publication No. (OS) 77–0004. Washington, D.C., U.S. Government Printing Office, 1977.

59. Due process for minors "voluntarily" committed to mental institutions: does father know best? *Southern Illinois Law Journal* 1980:171–190.

60. McCollum AT, Schwartz AH: Pediatric research hospitalization: its meaning to parents. *Pediat Res* 3:199–204, 1969.

61. Schoeman F: Protecting intimate relationships: children's competence and children's rights. *IRB* 4(6):1–6, 1982.

62. Vestal RE, Lawton MP, Ostfeld AM: Do elderly research subjects need special protections? *IRB* 2(8):5–8, 1980.

63. Bach-y-Rita G: The prisoner as an experimental subject. *JAMA* 229:45–46, 1974.

64. Kaimowitz v. Michigan Department of Mental Health, Civil Action 73–19434-AW (Wayne County, Mich., Cir. Ct. 1973), in Brooks AD: *Law, Psychiatry and the Mental Health System*. Boston, Little Brown, 1974, pp. 902–921.

65. Burt RA: Why we should keep prisoners from the doctors. *Hastings Center Report* 5(1):25–34, 1975.

66. Martin DC, Arnold JD, Zimmerman TF, et al.: Human subjects in clinical research—a report of three studies. *N Engl J Med* 279:1426–1431, 1968.

67. National Commission for the Protection of Human Subjects of Biomedical and Behavioral Research: *Research Involving Prisoners: Report and Recommendations*. DHEW Publication No. (OS) 76–131, Washington, D.C., U.S. Government Printing Office, 1976.

68. 21 Code of Federal Regulations §§ 50.40–50.48 (1984).

69. Sun M: Inmates sue to keep research in prisons. *Science* 212:650–651, 1981.

70. United States Department of Health, Education and Welfare, Food and Drug Administration: Protection of human subjects: prisoners used as research subjects; reproposal of regulations. *Federal Register* 46:61666–61671, December 18, 1981.

71. Murphy JG: Therapy and the problem of autonomous consent. *Int J Law Psychiatry* 2:415–430, 1979.

12

Fulfilling the Underlying Purpose of Informed Consent

To a great extent the underlying purposes of informed consent in research settings resemble those in the treatment situation. From a deontologic perspective, informed consent allows subjects to make meaningful decisions about participation in research projects. From a consequentialist point of view, informed consent is a means of reducing inequalities of knowledge and power in the researcher-subject relationship, thus increasing the cooperation and compliance of subjects. Increased knowledge also enhances patients' abilities to make decisions that will protect them from unwanted and undesirable intrusions on bodily integrity, perhaps of even greater importance here than in treatment settings, because of the sorry history of abuses inflicted on research subjects.

12.1 Subject and Researcher—A Divergence of Interests

As great as the similarities are, the differences are equally great. In treatment settings, as already noted, clinicians and patients are presumed to share the same goal: promoting patients' health. They may disagree over the means, but a general identity of interests is ordinarily the rule. Fried calls this confluence of interests the principle of personal care. "The traditional concept of the physician's relation to his patient is one of unqualified fidelity to that patient's health. He may certainly not do anything that would impair the patient's health and he must do everything in his ability to further it" (1, pp. 50–51). The essence of this principle is that physicians will not allow any other considerations to impinge on their decisions as to what measures are in patients' best interests.

Since the goal of scientific investigation is the production of generalizable knowledge, not primarily the promotion of individual health, there is at least the potential for a divergence of interests between subject and researcher (and for ambivalence on the part of the clinician-researcher). Steps taken to protect the generalizability of the data may conflict with the maximization of benefit to the individual subject (2). Therefore in research contexts—even in so-called therapeutic research, where treatment is intended to benefit the individual subject as well as produce generalizable knowledge—confluence of interests cannot be assumed. The need to take this conflict into account in the decisionmaking process is largely responsible for the differences between consent to research and to treatment.

The most striking potential for researcher-subject conflict of interest occurs in research that tests the relative efficacy of therapeutic interventions. A number of commentators have noted that modern scientific techniques are often responsible for actualizing this potential for conflict (1, pp. 47–78; 2–5). The clearest example of the problem is randomized assignment to experimental groups. Ordinarily, treatments are determined by patients' physicians based on individualized considerations of what would be most likely to help a particular patient. This process is short-circuited in controlled clinical trials by randomization, an important tool for minimizing bias in group assignment. The use of randomization is usually justified on the basis that controlled studies are only undertaken when researchers do not have conclusive evidence that one treatment is superior to the other (6). Thus, although clinician-researchers may be surrendering to the randomization process the right to select a treatment for their patients, and patients may be surrendering the benefit of that selection, it is argued that the patients do not suffer in this regard since they are going to be assigned to one of a number of equivalent treatments, as well as can be determined.

This argument fails to take into account, that, as some believe, existing knowledge does sometimes provide a reason to favor one treatment over another. *Investigators* may be impressed, for example, by the potential of a new medication that has had only uncontrolled trials, and thus be led to undertake a controlled comparison. An experienced *clinician* in such a situation might simply use the innovative drug, even though no scientifically adequate data exist supporting it. Besides such a general belief that one treatment might be superior, a clinician may have reason to believe a given treatment would be preferable for a particular patient. This belief may be based on a pattern of familial response to treatment, idiosyncratic elements of the patient's presentation, or the patient's own past experience with similar treatments. Subjects entering clinical trials lose the putative benefit of this informed speculation on their behalf, perhaps one of the most valued aspects of the doctor-patient relationship.

Subjects in randomized trials also lose the right to select among treatments which, even if their main effects are identical, may have significantly different side effects. Or they may lose the ability to trade off potential efficacy in main effect against the severity of side effects. Treatment for breast cancer is the most frequently offered example here (7; 8, pp. 90–103, 175–184). To avoid the disfigurement of a radical mastectomy, a woman may be willing to take a chance on a procedure that may be (but is not proven) less effective, and is certainly less mutilative. This power to take chances is lost when neither physician nor subject plays a role in deciding on treatment. Such a situation may further enhance feelings of helplessness in a hospitalized or seriously ill patient.

The ethics of randomization, largely in connection with these concerns, have become a matter of considerable controversy. The debate tends to overshadow similar issues raised by other aspects of scientific methodology. The use of placebos and nontreatment control groups also removes from subjects and their physicians the power to choose some well-considered, if imperfect, treatment over no treatment at all. In double-blind procedures, both patient-subjects and clinicians are kept in the dark about which group patients have been assigned to and what treatment they are receiving. These procedures are considered essential to preventing bias in treatment or evaluation. In these situations subjects are at risk when information is unavailable to help physicians monitor a clinical course or diagnose adverse reactions (4).

The constraints of a scientific protocol—the document that sets down what therapeutic interventions are and are not permissible in the conduct of a particular study—may also compromise individual decision making. In ordinary practice physicians might decide to raise or lower the dose of a medication, discharge a patient from the hospital, or add or delete adjunctive treatments. The rigidities of a protocol may limit a physician's ability to take these steps, regardless of patients' desires—short of dropping patients from the study, which neither physicians nor patients may want to do (2, 4–5). Entering a patient-subject into a protocol may also tend to freeze that patient's diagnosis, inhibiting refinement of the physician's conclusions, if they might lead to the patient being dropped from a study. Despite these considerations, when a prospective subject is adequately informed about the alternatives to participation, the relative risks and benefits within and outside of the experimental protocol, and the existence of randomized assignment and other constraints placed on patients and physicians by the research protocol, and voluntarily agrees to be a subject under these conditions, the losses associated with clinical research are ethically acceptable.

The potential for conflicts in research lacking therapeutic intent is less noticeable, but equally serious. Researchers and subjects may differ on the degree of risk that is advisable, with subjects being more risk averse. Although from an objective standpoint no doctor-patient relationship exists, and thus the principle of personal care may be thought not to apply, the subjects may not take this view. They may assume that physicians or scientists would never take measures that might endanger research subjects, and thus rely too much on the researchers to avoid risks. Researchers will be torn between the desire to live up to this expectation and the need to implement their protocol, which may involve the imposition of some degree of risk. Here again, the interests of researchers and their subjects are not identical.

Given these conflicts of interests, decision making about research must go one step beyond decision making about treatment.

In addition to disclosure of the nature, purpose, risks, and benefits of an intervention, along with the alternatives, decision making about research should involve a clarification of the differences between treatment and research, particularly the compromises of the principle of personal care that may have to be made. A focus and emphasis different from that of the treatment setting is required.

Many commentators have felt an uneasiness about violations of personal care (though they may not have used that term) inherent in much research. They have been led to suggest an additional goal of informed consent in research. The philosopher Hans Jonas, for example, expressed distress at the possibility that research subjects may come to be seen as manipulable means to researchers' ends rather than persons whose interests represent ends in themselves (9). The only corrective he saw to this problem is "such authentic identification [by the subject] with the cause that it is the subject's as well as the researcher's cause—whereby his role in its service is not just permitted by him, but *willed*. . . . [T]he appeal for volunteers should seek this free and generous endorsement, the appropriation of the research purpose into the person's own scheme of ends." Ramsey, a theologian and ethicist, has reached a similar conclusion—that it is only "men's capacity to become joint adventurers in a common cause [that] makes possible a consent to enter into the relation of patient to physician or of subject to investigator. This means that *partnership* is a better word than *contract* in conceptualizing the relation between patient and physician or between subject and investigator" (10, pp. 5–6).

Jonas and Ramsey, whose thoughts have profoundly influenced contemporary discussions of the ethics of research, seek to heal the conflict of interests by having the subject and investigator, like the physician and patient, work together toward a common goal. The means they envision for achieving this commonality involves a sufficiently detailed explanation of the research that the subject can willingly identify with and share the researchers' motivations—that is, a thorough informed consent. Although the worthiness of this goal is widely accepted and it may represent a valid ideal to strive for, it is probably unattainable in most circumstances. Besides, talking about common goals may obscure real conflicts of interests and thus complicate and confuse the decisionmaking pro-

242 CONSENT TO RESEARCH

cess. For example, the subject cannot be as single-mindedly devoted to the acquisition of data as the researcher when the subject alone takes the risk of discomfort, injury, or even death, and the researcher's career is being built on the data. Clarity may be enhanced by pointing to differences where they exist rather than papering them over with talk of a complete commonality of concerns. The requirement for informed consent provides a means of assuring an opportunity for conversation between investigators and prospective subjects. This opportunity should be used to explore not only matters included under the usual categories (risks, benefits, alternatives) but other matters of interest to potential subjects in deciding whether or not to participate in research.

12.2 Problems

Clarification of the research situation so that potential subjects can participate meaningfully in the decisionmaking process is a problematic task. Obstacles can arise in four areas: the investigator, the subject, the structure of the decisionmaking process, and communication of the necessary information.

The Investigator

Investigators' behavior remains an important stumbling block to a meaningful decisionmaking process. To some extent, investigators' failure to implement the doctrine of informed consent stems from a failure to assimilate its basic rationales. Appelbaum and Roth have found that of 17 investigators who worked with human subjects roughly half believed in the importance of informed consent as an ethical or practical principle, and the others rejected it as unattainable or as an unwarranted intrusion on the conduct of research (11).

Some researchers who hold negative views of the idea of informed consent believe that so much influence is exercised by the investigator over subjects that any attempt by them to protect their own interest, independent of the investigator, is meaningless (12). The subject has no alternative but to trust in the beneficence of the physician-investigator and the medical profession in general.

Other critics believe that neither patients in treatment nor subjects in research are really able to understand the information necessary to an informed decision (13,14). Garnham, for example, claimed on the basis of his experience with 41 volunteers that no one without medical training was able to acquire sufficient understanding of the risks of the research he conducted (14). Ingelfinger has argued similarly that without medical background to place risks and benefits into perspective, the result is what he calls informed but uneducated consent (13). This point of view has been challenged by studies showing that research subjects can be helped to understand a project's risks and benefits (15).

Researchers' resistance to informed consent can also result from a concern that the consent process (as they practice it—usually along the lines of the event model) inhibits and biases the recruitment of research subjects. Just as the application of informed consent in clinical situations often involves a delicate balance between autonomy and health values, so its application to research involves a potential conflict with the investigator's commitment to generating new knowledge. Investigators have obligations not only to their subjects but also to the disciplines they are trained in and to those who commit funds and other resources to the research.

Whether or not informed consent genuinely hinders research is unclear. One reported attempt to conduct a randomized trial of cancer chemotherapy was stymied by subjects' refusals to agree to randomization when they were informed that it would be employed (16). Another large national chemotherapy trial accrued subjects so slowly when using a standard consent procedure that its completion was threatened. The study was completed only when a controversial technique was used that allowed prerandomization without explicit consent for subjects assigned to the control group (17). Three groups have reported that patient-subjects who consented to psychiatric research were markedly different from the patient population as a whole. Spohn and Fitzpatrick have convincingly linked at least part of that variance to the consent process (18–20). Concerns have also been reported that informed consent may alter the nature of research results. One study has found that subjects who received information about drug side effects frequently were able to break the double-blind in a placebo-controlled study (21). Several psychological experiments have demonstrated differences in subject response based on whether or not disclosure had previously been made as part of the consent process (22).

Other studies have shown no difference in response rates to questionnaires or in willingness to participate in research because of the informed consent requirement (23–25). There is also substantial evidence that volunteer subjects are always somewhat different than the population they are drawn from (26, pp. 8–120). Moreover, the genuine cooperation a researcher obtains only from a subject who genuinely feels committed to the research may well offset much of the subtle undercutting of research that is of such concern.

Whether or not subject recruitment is adversely affected, however, the refusal of potential subjects to participate in a research project, even to the point of the project having to be abandoned, is entirely consistent with the nature of a democratic society. The scheme adopted by DHHS for the regulation of research is a two-step process. It requires, in effect, approval both by a panel of the investigators' peers and by potential research subjects. Peer approval (that is, by the IRB) is merely conditional. It allows the researcher to begin to approach potential subjects. Their subsequent approval is also required before the research may be undertaken. In other words, IRB approval permits the research to be undertaken on the condition that individual subjects agree to participate. Without IRB approval, individual subjects cannot even be approached for participation. On the other hand, there is nothing implicit in approval by the IRB (or a federal funding agency), that a research project must, or even should, be undertaken. Approval means only that it *may* be, assuming the willingness of individual subjects to participate. Whatever license researchers have to do research is a license to do research on *willing* subjects only. Investigators are no more entitled to complete a research project on unwilling subjects than noninvestigator physicians are to practice a proved therapy on unwilling patients.

Even investigators who acknowledge the desirability of informed consent, however, may find it difficult not to allow the boundary between research and therapeutic functions to be blurred (5,27). Investigators may experience discomfort with the necessary compromise of personal care in research settings. One study investigated physicians' reasons for not entering eligible patients in a randomized clinical trial of surgery for breast cancer (17). The trial had difficulties maintaining a steady rate of recruitment. Sixty-six of 91 surgeons who participated as coinvestigators failed to enroll all eligible patients in the research project. Among the reasons they gave for not seeking the consent of potential subjects were concern with the doctor-patient relationship in a randomized clinical trial (73 percent), trouble with informed consent (38 percent), conflict between physician as clinician and as scientist (18 percent), and feelings of personal responsibility if treatments were proved to be of unequal efficacy (8 percent).

In addition to having problems acknowledging conflicts between the roles of researcher and clinician, investigators often have difficulty discussing with a patient-subject their own uncertainty about the best treatment. Ironically, that very uncertainty is what motivates and legitimates a research study—there would be no need to conduct it if the best treatment were already known. Katz has argued that physicians are systematically trained to avoid discussing uncertainty with patients (8, pp. 165–206), despite demonstrations that uncertainty may be the single most important concept for both patients and physicians to grasp in all medical encounters, not just medical research (28, pp. 54–84). In the study of the problematic breast cancer protocol, 23 percent of surgeons who failed to enroll all eligible patients offered dislike of open discussions about uncertainty as a reason for their behavior (17).

Investigators' discomfort about informed consent can substantially affect the way in which consent is obtained. Studies of researchers' actual practices are rare. Some observational studies have suggested that members of the research team can underplay, distort, or even conceal information that would ordinarily be considered important in disclosure prior to obtaining consent (3; 29, pp. 190–192). Some investigators avoid the term research altogether and describe instead the aspects of the study that might benefit the individual subject (3). A study of the FDA's audit process for research subject to its oversight provides an estimate of the frequency of such problems. Of 964 routine audits conducted from 1977 to 1983, "problems with patient consent" were detected in 465 (48 percent) of the projects (30). A significant increase in the frequency of problems with consent has occurred since the current, more detailed revision of the FDA regulations governing informed consent was issued in 1981, from 39 to 61 percent of the deficiencies identified (31). Forty-two investigators were actually disciplined by the FDA for scientific misconduct between July 1977 and February 1983. Of the 41 on whom data was available, 18 (44 percent) were cited for "failure to obtain informed consent." These findings may actually understate the gravity of the problem. The FDA focuses its investigations on an audit of consent forms. Situations in which subjects signed seemingly adequate forms but were not given adequate oral explanations or opportunities to ask questions and have them answered would have gone unnoticed.

The Subjects

Subjects are not always comfortable with the goals of informed consent either. For example, patient-subjects in four psychiatric research projects voiced strong convictions that investigators were committed to acting solely in their best interests. This belief of patient-subjects that even in a research setting the principle of personal care will still apply has been called the therapeutic misconception (2). When not given information about how treatment decisions would be made, subjects fabricated reasonable-sounding explanations that placed their therapeutic interests first. Even when information was offered about the procedures that would be employed (e.g., randomization, double-blind, placebos), many subjects failed to acknowledge what they had heard, to apply it to their own circumstances, or to admit that the procedures served any interests other than their personal care.

One subject, for example, volunteered the information that assignment to active medication or placebo would be on a random basis. When she was asked directly how her own medication would be selected, she said she had no idea. She then added, "I hope it isn't by chance," and suggested that each subject would probably receive the medication needed. Given the conflict between her earlier use of the word random and her current explanation, the issue was pursued. She was asked what her understanding of random was. Her definition was entirely appropriate: "By lottery, by chance, one patient who comes in gets one thing and the next patient gets the next thing." She then began to wonder out loud if this procedure was being used in the current study. Ultimately, she concluded that it was not. Subjects apparently had been so socialized by their previous experiences in medical care settings, in which their expectation of personal care was realistic, that they were unable to adapt to the different norms of the research setting.

This type of therapeutic orientation toward research has been demonstrated in a wide variety of circumstances. For example, when a group of fourteen psychiatric outpatients were told they would be given sugar pills rather than pills containing active medication, about half of them believed that the pills contained active medication, and only three patients reported no doubts that the pills were placebos (32). The researchers attributed this response to "the force of prior experiences, which at times induced patients to disregard or to disbelieve the doctor's assertion" that no active medication was being given. These subjects' therapeutic misconception appeared to be firmly grounded in their difficulty with distinguishing previous treatment experiences from the current research setting.

The frequency of this confusion between therapeutic and research goals was confirmed by a study showing that 75 percent of patients in research projects at four Veterans Administration hospitals decided to participate because they expected the research to have a beneficial effect on their health (33). A survey of attitudes toward research in a combined sample of patients and the general public showed an interesting discrepancy in responses. When asked why people in general should participate in research, 69 percent of respondents cited benefit to society at large. Only 5 percent cited benefit to the subjects themselves. However, when asked why *they* might participate in a research project, 52 percent said they would do it to get the best medical care, and only 23 percent responded that they would do it to contribute to scientific knowledge (34). In another study, among patient-subjects on a psychiatric research ward, the largest group of patients expressed the idea that "research is therapy—a patient and his family often believe that a prestigious research center will be able to cure him when other therapies and hospitals have failed" (27,35). Similarly, subjects frequently interpreted the word research to mean "finding out more about me" or "researching how to treat me better," an entirely personalized and therapeutic understanding of the research endeavor (2).

The Structure of the Decisionmaking Process

Structural problems may also play a role in impeding the process of obtaining informed consent. Investigators often delegate the responsibility for informing and obtaining consent from potential subjects to subordinates who may be unable to clarify subjects' concerns. In a sample of 17 investigators, only 8 were ever directly involved in the disclosure and consent process, and only 4 were routinely involved throughout the disclosure (11). (In contrast, a study at four Veterans Administration hospitals revealed that 70 percent of 37 principal investigators *said* that they or a coinvestigator were responsible for obtaining consent [33]). Delegation of responsibility for informed consent to a junior person on the research team may not only demonstrate the investigator's belief that obtaining consent is of little consequence but also place the process in the hands of an individual with little understanding of the ethical issues involved. Further, a research assistant who is responsible for recruitment of subjects may feel pressure to obtain subjects' consent and thus be led to distort or omit significant information. One study has shown that investigators infrequently monitor the performance of their subordinates to whom they delegate this responsibility (11).

A second kind of structural problem relates to the inherent pressures on subjects as they decide whether or not to participate. Clearly it would be unethical to withhold an otherwise available treatment in an effort to coerce a patient into joining a research project. However, there are occasions when the desired treatment is only available as part of the research (e.g., when the research involves an investigational drug or a highly specialized procedure). To the extent that a goal of informed consent is an uncoerced choice, the intrinsically coercive character of a situation in which the desired treatment is only available as part of a protocol makes attainment of voluntary informed consent impossible. There simply is no way to avoid the existence of such situations. The degree and quality of limitation on free choice here is no greater than those encountered in everyday life, in which hard decisions and trade-offs must be made. The real danger is that patients in their eagerness to become subjects of the study in order to receive the restricted treatment will fail to attend to other information that might alter their assessment of the value of participation.

The Communication of Necessary Information

Difficulties in the communication of information can also form a barrier to the goals of informed consent. Complex research projects often require lengthy explanations of elements that are relevant to a potential subject's risk-benefit analysis. When committed to writing, the resulting consent forms often run several pages. Federal regulations governing the material that must appear on consent forms, including such items as whether treatment or compensation will be available if injuries occur, also contribute to the length of the forms. And subjects' comprehension of consent forms, and consequent willingness to participate, may be an inverse function of the forms' length (36). (See Chapter 9.)

What is true for consent forms probably holds for oral explanations as well. Studies are lacking in this regard. It seems likely that researchers' (often unconscious) addiction to jargon makes oral disclosure problematic for subjects. Simplification would probably increase the length of the explanation and reduce the amount subjects are able to comprehend.

12.3 A Reasonable Approach: Dispelling the Therapeutic Misconception

Obtaining informed consent to research requires good faith and some effort on the part of investigators. Neither the requirements of the law and relevant ethical codes nor the obstacles that commonly arise in the decisionmaking process prevent researchers from fulfilling the requirement of informed consent in a reasonable way.

Content of Disclosure

To some extent the decision about what information should be provided is more easily determined in research than in the purely therapeutic setting. Federal regulations (as outlined in Chapter 11), along with additional state and institutional requirements, specify in some detail the material that must be disclosed. In essence, the federal rules require disclosure of the fact that the nature and purpose of the procedures are experimental, the risks and benefits, the alternatives (in therapeutic situations), and ancillary information on such issues as confidentiality, compensation for injuries, and the right to withdraw from the study. Institutional requirements may supplement these items—for example, asking investigators to inform subjects of the source of funding of their research.

The specificity conveyed by the federal rules and their progeny is to a large extent spurious. Experienced investigators are aware that particularly in complex investigations, in which only a fraction of the available information can actually be disclosed, a large amount of discretion resides in the hands of researchers (and IRBs) to decide what need and need not be revealed. Since IRBs generally focus on written consent forms, ignoring the oral communication that ought occur as well, investigators have the further ability to shape the tone and substance of the oral disclosure either to underscore or undercut the material in the consent form (29).

Even when they are supportive of the goals of informed consent, researchers may be confused about what subjects need to know in order to make informed decisions. This confusion is accentuated by the fact that anyone intimately familiar with a topic has difficulty empathizing with the problems of understanding faced by a person unfamiliar with the field. Guidance in this regard has tended to take the form of admonitions to adhere to existing regulations, which—as we have seen—are of little assistance, or to engage the potential subject as a collaborator. The latter approach may only further confuse the investigator about what amount and level of material needs to be revealed.

A more focused approach derives from an awareness of the ways treatment and research differ. Taking this distinction as the conceptual core of disclosure provides a touchstone for investigators. Specifically, in covering the nature, purpose, overall risks and benefits, alternatives, and other specified disclosures required by the federal regulations and state statutes or common law, investigators can ask themselves whether their planned disclosure will help potential subjects comprehend the differences between what they would undergo in the research project and what they would obtain in ordinary clinical treatment. This approach is relevant even in research unlikely to have therapeutic benefit, since even here subjects are likely to extrapolate from the clinical setting, assuming that research procedures are intended to benefit them or at the least not to cause them harm. One subject in nontherapeutic research explained that he had joined a research project despite the possible consequences of severe liver damage because, he said, "Doctor, we know you wouldn't hurt us, and anyway the hospital wouldn't let you" (14).

The discussion between investigator and potential subject, and the consent form, should focus on the distinction between therapy and research. Where the research consists of a study of a therapy or therapies—such as comparison of an accepted therapy with an innovative therapy, or comparison of a therapy (accepted or innovative) and a placebo, or comparison of all three—the emphasis must be on the distinction between therapy and research on therapy. Where the potential subject could obtain a particular therapy either in the context of the study or outside the study, much of the information to be provided is the same as in the purely clinical setting. The distinctive features to be called to potential subjects' attention are the nature and purpose of the research, the risks and benefits of being a subject, and the available options for obtaining the same or different therapies outside of the research setting. In particular, potential subjects need to be told about those features of being a research subject that do not exist in ordinary therapy, such as the possible use of placebos or the selection of treatment by randomization.

Such an approach, for projects in which therapies are being employed, can proceed in the following way: After being told that they are being asked to participate in a research project, potential subjects can be informed that the procedures in the project differ from those of the clinical care they would ordinarily receive. "Because this is a research project," the investigator might say, "we will be doing some things differently from what we would do if we were simply treating you for your condition." The investigator can then describe what the research is designed to demonstrate and how it will be conducted, with special emphasis on the aspects that differ from ordinary clinical care.

Although many of the elements of research design that differ most significantly from ordinary treatment are based on sophisticated statistical and methodological principles, they can often be explained quite simply. Potential subjects could be told about randomization in this way: "You will receive one of the three treatments we discussed, but the one you receive will be selected by chance, not because we believe that one or the other will be better for you." About placebos: "Some subjects will be selected by chance to receive sugar pills that are not known to help the condition you have; this is done so we can find out whether the medications other patients get are really effective, or if many people with your condition would get better even with no active medication at all." About the use of protocols: "Ordinarily doctors change the amount of medication according to how their patients are doing. Here, in order to test the usefulness of the medications we are trying out, we will have to leave your dosage at the same level for four weeks—unless you suffer a severe reaction to it."

Once potential subjects have the distinctions between the research project and ordinary treatment clearly in mind, they can be told about the other risks of participation as well as the benefits to themselves and others that might derive from the research project. Care must also be taken to insure that subjects are informed of the risks and benefits of the underlying therapy or therapies on which research is being conducted, and to distinguish between the risks and benefits that arise from treatment in general, and risks and benefits that will accrue only as a result of participation in the project. The alternative of treatment outside a research protocol, if available, should be clearly outlined here, and the subject's right to elect a usual form of treatment or withdraw from the study at any time should be stressed. Finally, any additional information relevant to a particular project or required by regulations can be provided. The understanding of potential subjects should be assessed continually, and additional information provided to correct misperceptions or misunderstandings as they occur and are detected. Subjects can also be given an opportunity to ask questions about the material that has been presented.

This outline would be somewhat different for research in which no therapeutic methods were being employed that would benefit even some of the subjects. Yet, the basic idea that needs to be communicated is much the same and could be stated thus: "Our primary goal is to obtain information about the issue we are studying, not to benefit you in any way. This is true even though you may find participation interesting or educational." Purpose and procedures can then be described, again emphasizing the fact that the selection of various experimental conditions is being made for experimental reasons and not with beneficial intent. Risks can then also be reviewed.

As has been stated, what is important about the approach described here is the effort to underline in potential subjects' minds the differences between research and treatment, or in some cases the lack of overall therapeutic intent. The precise wording and even the order of the disclosure can vary considerably, depending on the nature of the research project, the preferences of the investigators, and the potential subjects' educational levels. In their efforts to convey these distinctions, physician–investigators must not lose sight of the fact that they are also obligated to adhere to the normal rules for obtaining informed consent that would prevail in the absence of a research protocol. That is, potential subjects must also be adequately informed of the risks, benefits, nature, and purpose of the investigated therapies themselves.

Deception in the process of recruiting research subjects is a technique frequently used in social psychological experiments, in an attempt to control the mindset subjects bring to the experimental situation (22). Outright deception, though permitted by current federal regulations and the ethical code of the American Psychological Association (37), has been the subject of considerable criticism. Leading opponents of the practice have charged that deception does not actually produce a naturalistic situation, and thus its putative advantages may be a sham (38). A hot debate rages over these contentions (39). It is also argued that in the long-term deception may have an adverse impact on the entire research enterprise because researchers will eventually be able to enlist only cynical, distrustful subjects and may forfeit public support for their research (38).

The most telling argument against deception is that it is disrespectful of persons. It serves the acquisition of knowledge while demeaning human dignity and is therefore simply incompatible with the underlying premise of informed consent, the entitlement of subjects to make knowing decisions about participation in research. Even were it proven effective, and its aftereffects mitigated completely by debriefing, deception still represents a serious intrusion on individual autonomy. Of course, subjects should have the freedom to consent to deception—that is, to agree knowingly to the researcher's withholding of some unspecified information from them. But complete deception cannot be justified within the framework of informed consent.

Disclosure as a Process

There are numerous benefits for both patients and physicians in a model that views consent as a process rather than an event. (See Chapter 8.) The same is true for investigators and subjects. Thus, the dialogue between investigator and potential subject outlined above need not proceed linearly or take place as a single event. Particularly when potential subjects are accessible for a period of time, as inpatients or students might be, discussions can take place on a number of occasions, and the intervening periods can allow subjects to integrate and reflect on the information provided and to formulate questions and focus concerns (40). A subject's agreement to participate in research, signified by signing a consent form, should not be seen as the end of the process. Questions will arise; information will be forgotten; new concerns may come to the fore. The subject's right to withdraw at any time is a reminder of the need to view informed consent as a continuing, interactive process, with consent in effect renewed each time an experimental procedure takes place.

A variety of devices can facilitate this process. Allowing potential subjects to review written material and ask questions about it at a later time, prior to obtaining formal consent, can be useful. Additional information can then be provided as needed. All written material should attempt to strike a reasonable balance between clarity and brevity. Testing the comprehension of a sample of persons with educational backgrounds similar to those in the subject pool may be of use. Consent forms, required in many research settings, can play a useful role in informing subjects but must not be allowed to dominate the process (41). (See Chapter 9.)

Our discussion has proceeded as if the principal investigator were the only person directly involved in obtaining informed consent. In many projects this involvement is impossible. For example, in large-scale epidemiologic surveys subjects may be recruited over a wide geographic area, and in projects with heavy subject flows, several subjects may be recruited simultaneously. It may simply be impossible for the investigators themselves to make time to obtain informed consent from all subjects. Thus, delegation of the responsibility inevitably occurs in many studies. This delegation is not necessarily bad, as long as investigators clearly communicate the importance of the process to the staff members responsible and assign the task only to persons who understand the ethical concerns underlying consent and who know enough about the projects to answer the questions likely to arise. Furthermore, staff should not be under such unreasonable pressures to meet subject quotas that they might be tempted to distort the disclosure process to attain that goal. The supervising investigators should obtain informed consent themselves at least a few times early in the course of a study, so as to become familiar with problems that may arise and better instruct their subordinates about them. Periodic checks on how informed consent is being obtained may be of use, too. This procedure would address the reported problems of investigators who have clear ideas about what kind of subject might be incompetent to consent to their study but have never communicated these ideas to the staff who must obtain consent, and have no awareness of how the issue is being handled in practice (11).

As desirable as investigator involvement is, in some cases it may be optimal for someone else to be involved in addition or instead. Particularly in research on therapeutic procedures where the investigator also acts as the subject's physician, there may be a strong tendency on the part of subjects to merge in their minds the goals of research and treatment. The investigators themselves may be unwilling or unable to help subjects identify the nontherapeutic aspects of the proposed research or the additional risks it might entail. When those risks are particularly great, there is ample justification for IRBs to require that investigators' explanations be supplemented by information from an uninvolved party. This person, while not injuring the researcher-subject relationship and not interfering with the communication of information that the investigator wishes to stress, can pay particular attention to the distinctions between treatment and research.

Balancing the Costs and Benefits

The approach to informed consent suggested here has costs and benefits. It seems reasonable to believe that the more clearly potential subjects understand the difference between research and treatment (and thus the additional risks they may incur from research participation) the more likely they may be to decline to participate in research. This phenomenon may slow down recruitment in some studies, bias samples, and perhaps prevent certain research altogether. No data are available to tell us how likely these consequences are, and some arguments exist against the underlying assumption. Some claim that subjects may be so impressed by the honesty and openness of investigators who reveal information that cuts against investigators' interests in recruiting subjects that they may decide to enroll in the study anyway on the grounds that the investigator is a person who can be trusted.

We are probably safe in assuming that some negative impact on subject recruitment is likely. Ought that cost to be tolerated? It may not be as great as is usually assumed. It may be mitigated by the alternatives to randomized clinical trials (the most problematic type of research project where consent is concerned) and the techniques for correcting for resulting biases statistically (7). What happens when these are not possible? Angell's response is to the point: "What can be done when nonrandomized designs are considered inadequate but randomization would be difficult because of patients' preferences for one treatment or the other? Not all problems have solutions. It simply may not be ethically possible to conduct a valid randomized clinical trial under these circumstances" (7). If our efforts to promote individual autonomy by allowing subjects to make informed decisions about participation may succeed only at the cost of slowing some scientific endeavors, that cost may simply have to be tolerated.

It would be wrong not to consider the potential benefits of an approach that emphasizes dispelling the therapeutic misconception. Well-informed patients may be more cooperative with research procedures and more willing to participate in later extensions of research projects. As Park and his colleagues noted, "Informing patients might be especially helpful in long term studies and follow-up studies in which patient cooperation would be facilitated by the patient's awareness of the significance of this participation not only for himself but for patients in the future. This kind of doctor-patient collaborative atmosphere would be conducive to the acceptance of arrangements in which patients could be called back or visited at home at predefined intervals" (42). For some types of research, subject cooperation may be a crucial determinant of success.

The advantages of having well-informed subjects are also clear when one considers what might happen if and when subjects discover that they have misunderstood the purposes of the study procedures and the degree of benefit to themselves. Subjects coming to such a realization during a study might drop out and thereby disrupt the conduct of the protocol. Subjects whose realization occurs only after the conclusion of a study may be left with anger and resentment against the researchers who they feel deceived them, even if their own desire to see research through therapeutic lenses contributed mightily to the deception. Such subjects will be unlikely ever again to consider research participation. As they tell their stories to sympathetic relatives and friends, they may contribute to a general perception that researchers treat patients as guinea pigs. The failure to distinguish between researchers and clinicians may contribute to a general perception that all physicians (or psychologists, sociologists, or scientists in general) cannot be trusted. Since most research is heavily dependent on public support—both for funding and participation as subjects—the spread of such perceptions may constitute a threat to the research enterprise as a whole more serious than the inability to perform a few studies because of a scarcity of available subjects.

Well-informed subjects, while recognizing the potential conflict between their interests and those of investigators, nonetheless realize to some extent the goal of shared objectives advocated by Jonas and Ramsey. Such subjects are likely to prove strong allies in the future. They may benefit from learning more about the conduct of research, and in special cases their knowing participation may even have beneficial effects on their behavior in other areas (43). Disclosure of the type suggested in this chapter may make things easier for some investigators as well. The guilt that has been observed among researchers, deriving from the recognition that they are acting in ways that may be contrary to subjects' best interests, can be mitigated by limiting involvement to subjects who are truly aware of the risks they are running (5,42).

A focus on dispelling the therapeutic misconception will lead to greater respect for subjects' autonomy, and perhaps more cooperative subjects as well.

References

1. Fried C: *Medical Experimentation: Personal Integrity and Social Policy.* New York, American Elsevier, 1974.

2. Appelbaum PS, Roth LH, Lidz CW: The therapeutic misconception: informed consent in psychiatric research. *Int J Law Psychiatry* 5:319–329, 1982.

3. Benson PR, Roth LH, Winslade WJ: Informed consent in psychiatric research: preliminary findings from an ongoing investigation. *Soc Sci Med* 20:133–1341, 1985.

4. Howard J, Friedman L: Protecting the scientific integrity of a clinical trial: some ethical dilemmas. *Clin Pharmacol Ther* 29:561–569, 1981.

5. Epstein RS, Janowsky DS: Research on the psychiatric ward: the effects on conflicting priorities. *Arch Gen Psychiatry* 21:455–463, 1969.

6. Levine RJ: *Ethics and Regulation of Clinical Research.* Baltimore, Urban and Schwarzenberg, 1981, pp. 126–129.

7. Angell M: Patients' preferences in randomized clinical trials. *N Engl J Med* 310:1385–1387, 1984.

8. Katz J: *The Silent World of Doctor and Patient.* New York, Free Press, 1984.

9. Jonas H: Philosophical reflections on experimenting with human subjects, in Freund PA (ed.), *Experimentation with Human Subjects.* New York, Braziller, 1970.

10. Ramsey P: *The Patient as Person.* New Haven, Yale University Press, 1977.

11. Appelbaum PS, Roth LH: The structure of informed consent in psychiatric research. *Behavioral Sciences and the Law* 1:9–19, 1983.

12. Beecher HK: Consent in clinical experimentation: myth and reality. *JAMA* 195:124–125, 1966.

13. Ingelfinger FJ: Informed (but uneducated) consent. *N Engl J Med* 287:465–466, 1972.

14. Garnham JC: Some observations on informed consent in non-therapeutic research. *J Med Ethics* 1:138–145, 1975.

15. Howard JM, DeMets D, and the BHAT Research Group: How informed

is informed consent? The BHAT experience. *Controlled Clinical Trials* 2:287–303, 1981.

16. Lacher MJ: Physicians and patients as obstacles to a randomized trial. *Clin Res* 26:375–379, 1978.

17. Taylor KM, Margolese RG, Soskolne CL: Physicians' reasons for not entering eligible patients in a randomized clinical trial for breast cancer. *N Engl J Med* 310:1363–1367, 1984.

18. Schubert DSP, Patterson MB, Miller FT, et al.: Informed consent as a source of bias in clinical research. *Psychiatr Res* 12:313–320, 1984.

19. Spohn HE, Fitzpatrick T: Informed consent and bias in samples of schizophrenic subjects at risk for drug withdrawal. *J Abnormal Psychol* 89:79–92, 1980.

20. Edlund MJ, Craig TJ, Richardson MA: Informed consent as a form of volunteer bias. *Am J Psychiatry* 142:624–627, 1985.

21. Brownell KD, Stunkard AJ: The double-blind in danger: untoward consequences of informed consent. *Am J Psychiatry* 139:1487–1489, 1982.

22. Adair JG, Dushenko, TW, Lindsay RCL: Ethical regulations and their impact on research practice. *Am Psychologist* 40:59–72, 1985.

23. Singer E: Informed consent: consequences for response rate and response quality in social surveys. *American Sociological Review* 43:144–162, 1978.

24. McLean PD: The effect of informed consent on the acceptance of random treatment assignment in a clinical population. *Behavior Ther* 11:129–133, 1980.

25. Kokes RF, Fremouw W, Strauss JS: Lost subjects: source of bias in clinical research? *Arch Gen Psychiatry* 34:1363–1365, 1977.

26. Rosenthal R, Rosnow RL: *The Volunteer Subject*. New York, Wiley, 1975.

27. Jacobs L, Kotin J: Fantasies of psychiatric research. *Am J Psychiatry* 128:1074–1080, 1972.

28. Bursztajn H, Feinbloom RI, Hamm RM, et al.: *Medical Choices, Medical Chances: How Patients, Families, and Physicians Can Cope with Uncertainty*. New York, Delacorte, 1981.

29. Lidz C, Meisel A, Zerubavel E, et al.: *Informed Consent: A Study of Decisionmaking in Psychiatry*. New York, Guilford, 1984.

30. Shapiro MF, Charrow RP: Scientific misconduct in investigational drug trials. *N Engl J Med* 312:731–736, 1985.

31. 21 Code of Federal Regulations §§ 50.1–50.27, 56.101–56.124 (1984).

32. Park LC, Covi L: Nonblind placebo trial: an exploration of neurotic patients' responses to placebo when its inert content is disclosed. *Arch Gen Psychiatry* 12:336–345, 1965.

33. Riecken HW, Ravich R: Informed consent to biomedical research in Veterans Administration hospitals. *JAMA* 248:344–348, 1982.

34. Cassileth BR, Lusk EJ, Miller DS, et al.: Attitudes toward clinical trials among patients and the public. *JAMA* 248:968–970, 1982.

35. Leigh V: Attitudes and fantasy themes of patients on a psychiatric research unit. *Arch Gen Psychiatry* 32:598–601, 1975.

36. Epstein LC, Lasagna L: Obtaining informed consent—form or substance. *Arch Intern Med* 123:682–688, 1969.

37. American Psychological Association: Ethical principles in the conduct of research with human participants. Washington, D.C., APA, 1973.

38. Baumrind D: Research using intentional deception: ethical issues revisited. *Am Psychologist* 40:165–174, 1985.

39. Baron RA: The "Costs of Deception" revisited: an openly optimistic rejoinder. *IRB* 3(1):8–10, 1981.

40. Carpenter WT: A new setting for informed consent. *Lancet* 1:500–501, 1974.

41. Lidz CW, Roth LH: The signed form—informed consent? in Boruch RF, Ross J, Cecil JS (eds.), *Solutions to Legal and Ethical Problems in Applied Social Research*. New York, Academic Press, 1981.

42. Park LC, Covi L, Uhlenhuth EH: Effects of informed consent on research patients and study results. *J Nerv Ment Dis* 145:349–357, 1967.

43. Siris SG, Docherty JP, McGlashan TH: Intrapsychic structural effects of psychiatric research. *Am J Psychiatry* 136:1567–1571, 1979.

V

ADVANCING INFORMED CONSENT

13

An Agenda for the Future

The cornerstone of our approach to informed consent is the belief that the right of patients to participate in making their own medical decisions, usually called the right to autonomy in decision making, is a moral value worth promoting. When medical care is required, patients should be met by physicians' openness and willingness to present and discuss a variety of options, with the clear understanding that patients can play a role, if they desire, in shaping the ultimate decision. Our instinctive assumption that most patients would endorse this approach was confirmed by a large-scale study sponsored by the President's Commission (1). Patients do want to know about and have the option of influencing the nature of their medical care. Our society's deep-seated traditions of respect for the integrity of the individual reinforce the importance of protecting patients' interests in the medical decisionmaking process.

Legal initiatives by themselves are insufficient to accomplish these results. (See Chapter 7.) The legal rules governing informed consent operate at a level of generality that makes it difficult for physicians to take them into account in dealing with patients. Surveys have revealed that most physicians are completely ignorant of the operative standard for disclosure in their state (1).

More significantly, however, the medical setting seems relatively impervious to regulation. Physicians and administrators have control over the structure of medical care and over the content of physician-patient interactions. Regardless of the law of informed consent, if the structure of hospital and office practice provides negligible opportunities for doctor-patient communication, little disclosure or shared decision making will occur. If physicians are resistant to the moral imperatives of informed consent, tinkering with standards of disclosure is unlikely to affect their behavior. Physicians, other health care personnel, and their attorneys are sufficiently imaginative and in control of the situation to devise means of defeating the intent of most legal regulation, perhaps even masking their response as mechanical compliance with its mandates.

For three decades legal stratagems have been employed to compel physicians, and now other health-care professionals, to respect their patients as persons with the right to know about and help shape their medical care. Although some changes have occurred in doctor-patient interactions, we believe that in the long run attempts to force people to respect others are doomed to failure. One can create a framework in which respect can develop. One can even compel behavior similar to what would occur were respect to exist. But respect is so personal a characteristic that it either flows from a genuine source, or not at all. In essence, this is the paradox in which the law of informed consent has been caught. The legal requirements have gone as far as they can. The framework for respect has been created and codes of behavior have been prescribed. And that has not been enough.

We do not believe that the legal requirements for informed consent should be dismantled, nor that they should be materially revised. Such action could not but be interpreted by physicians and other caregivers as a signal that informed consent is no longer to be taken seriously. But for further progress we must look elsewhere. Even granting the unlikely assumption that elements of physicians' overt behavior could be controlled by law, it is clear that attitudinal change must be accomplished by different means. Physicians must come to accept the values underlying informed consent before they will behave accordingly.

A change in attitudes can only be brought about by systematic efforts to educate physicians. A two-pronged approach will be required. First, physicians should be exposed to the ethical principles behind the idea of informed consent, so that they can come to understand and, most importantly, internalize them. Second, physicians must be persuaded that a model for the implementation of informed consent exists that does not compromise, but enhances, the physician-patient relationship and the delivery of medical care. Physicians must come to believe that the interests of autonomy and health can be reconciled in a manner that does not do unacceptable damage to the latter. We have attempted in this book to conceptualize and delineate such a model, which we termed the process model of informed consent. The question remains how both the values and the model can be communicated to physicians.

As a first step, students in medical and other health professional schools must be taught to recognize that each party brings unique attributes and capacities to bear on medical decision making. Patients' contributions to the process are not inferior to those of physicians, but merely different in kind, and of irreplaceable importance, insofar as they best embody patients' systems of values. Students must learn the ethical theories of autonomy. Their anxiety about performing as clinicians, along with their nascent sense of professional identity, may make it difficult for them to accept the need to share information and decision making with patients. Students should be encouraged to place themselves in the position of patients, a role that is still more familiar to them than that of clinicians. They will also need to review the legal foundations of the doctor-patient relationship, along with the clinical principles— now taught in many medical schools—on which effective physician-patient interaction rests.

Others before us have emphasized the importance, in achieving the goals of informed consent, of such education (2, pp. 150–154; 3, pp. 135–149). We believe that the magnitude of the task has been underestimated, and implementation has barely begun.

Discussions of informed consent issues in the preclinical years are of use, but must be supplemented by hands-on training in the process model during clinical rotations. Students should be taught how to communicate information, facilitate patient participation, and handle questions of impaired competency and voluntariness. They should receive feedback on their performance in this area, just as in other aspects of delivering medical care.

Some medical and other health professional schools have begun to revise their curricula in keeping with these ideas. Many—probably most—have not. But it would be an enormous error to believe that efforts restricted to the years of formal schooling will be sufficient to change the attitudes of health professionals. Instruction at this level merely sets the stage for more crucial intervention later on. The initial years of functioning with responsibility in a clinical setting—for physicians, the years of residency—have the most powerful influence on enduring patterns of professional behavior. It is during these years that physicians learn how to interact with patients. They model their behavior on that of their seniors and supervisors, and they experiment with a variety of approaches on their own. The benefits of years of excellent medical school instruction can be lost in a few months if residents' early steps in the right direction are not properly reinforced.

Currently, physicians in residency training learn from what they see around them that informed consent is a nuisance, an alien imposition of the legal system that must be tolerated, because of possible legal consequences, but can be dealt with in relatively mechanical ways, such as making sure patients sign consent forms before major procedures. They learn that patients must be listened to early in the evaluation process because they may be an important source of valuable diagnostic information, but that once the physician has made a diagnosis and decided on a plan of action, the patient's role goes no further than *pro forma* ratification of the physician's choice. They are taught by example that a system of medical care that minimizes doctor-patient interaction is acceptable, and that given economic pressures—such as fixed reimbursements for diagnosis-related groups—such a system may even be desirable.

There is no hope for informed consent as an ethical doctrine or even as a meaningful set of legal rules unless this situation changes. During residency training (and equivalent periods for nonphysician health-care personnel), physicians must be taught that patients have a legitimate and important role to play in shaping decisions about their care, and that this role can be fulfilled in a reasonable manner. This teaching can only be accomplished by a combination of direct instruction and indirect modeling both of the importance of these attitudes and of the behavior that facilitates patients' playing this role. Since relatively few physicians today incorporate such an approach in their own practices, a small cadre of teachers will have to train a larger group of instructors for this purpose. At first, time for teaching this approach will need to be set aside, despite the already heavy time pressures on residents. As graduates of the initial years of teaching themselves assume supervisory roles, greater reliance could be placed on having residents model their supervisors' behavior, with formal didactic sessions taking a subordinate role.

One should not, of course, write off the physicians in practice today, who will be determining the shape of our medical care well into the next century. Remedial programs (though physicians might understandably resist such a designation) for physicians who have never been exposed to the idea of a collaborative approach to the doctor-patient relationship should be organized. It is likely, as well, that when older physicians are exposed to the new ideas and practices their juniors have learned (assuming the success of the other levels of training), their behavior will begin to change. Nonetheless, the difficulty of altering established patterns of interaction should not be underestimated. The primary emphasis must be on insuring that another generation of physicians and other health-care personnel does not perpetuate the current unsatisfactory situation.

In addition to renewed educational efforts, changes now under way in how health-care delivery is organized—especially the trend toward prepaid medical care—might enhance the prospects for the realization of the genuine spirit of informed consent. These new health-care structures are premised to an increasing extent on ideas about preventive medicine and holistic health. Whether for ideological or economic reasons, they treat patients less as objects to be ministered to and more as full-fledged participants in decisions about their health. We may soon begin to see an expansion of innovative attempts at patient education, including greater use of nurses and other health-care personnel whose time is less expensive than physicians'. At the same time, there is a real danger that shortsighted attempts to lower immediate health-care costs may lead some organized care settings to even further restrict patient contact with health professionals.

What are we likely to gain from an effort to improve the training of clinicians in regard to informed consent, considering the time, money, and energy it will cost? To be realistic, our expectations must be somewhat circumscribed. We consider utopian the idea that all patients could fully understand the risks, benefits, and alternatives recommended by their physicians. We doubt that all patients, or even a substantial majority, will want to make their decisions about their medical care singlehandedly—if they even could do so. Many patients may not want to participate in the decisionmaking process at all. How many decisions will be made differently is admittedly unclear.

None of these conclusions negate, in our eyes, the value of encouraging physicians to conform to the model of doctor-patient interactions and the process of medical decision making described in this book. The value is less that it will alter the outcome of the decisionmaking process than that it will change the nature of the process itself. Patients will be treated with the respect they deserve as autonomous individuals. To the extent that they make the effort to comprehend the information provided (and, of course, reasonable attempts should be made to insure that the information is inherently comprehensible) and wish to participate, they will have the opportunity to do so. Even if they do not make the effort to grasp all of the data and its implications, or if they willingly cede decisionmaking authority to their physicians, they will still be treated as if the right to do otherwise is theirs, which in fact it is.

The effects of such a change are unpredictable, but let us speculate on just how far-reaching they could become. When people are treated differently, they begin to respond differently. Patients who are treated as respected partners in medical care may begin to behave with a new level of responsibility. They may take more initiative to maintain their own health, comply with agreed-on regimens, and provide important information to their physicians. As active decision makers rather than passive recipients of care, they may acknowledge that they deserve partial credit for good results, but also partial blame for results that turn out poorly. A lessening of the tendency to blame physicians for adverse outcomes may reduce the desire to seek legal remedies through the malpractice system. A greater recognition of the degree of uncertainty in medical treatment, which can be expected to flow from a discussion of alternative courses of treatment, may also have the same effect.

The positive side effects of the model we have presented are of course entirely speculative. Yet they may serve as a counterweight to the speculative disadvantages commonly given credence in medical circles: increased numbers of refusals of needed treatment, heightened anxiety among patients, and, above all, the wasteful use of precious medical time. Even if these putative advantages were not to materialize, however, we would still urge adoption of our model. Informed consent—and by that we refer both to the idea of informed consent and the resulting legal requirements—is important because it ratifies and protects the uniqueness of the individual patient. For us, and by now we hope for the reader of this book, that is justification enough.

References

1. Harris L, and associates: Views of informed consent and decisionmaking: parallel surveys of physicians and the public, in President's Commission for the Study of Ethical Problems in Medicine and Biomedical and Behavioral Research, *Making Health Care Decisions: The Ethical and Legal Implications of Informed Consent in the Patient-Practitioner Relationship.* Vol. 2, *Appendix.* Washington, D.C., U.S. Government Printing Office, 1982.

2. President's Commission for the Study of Ethical Problems in Medicine and Biomedical and Behavioral Research: *Making Health Care Decisions: The Ethical and Legal Implications of the Patient-Practitioner Relationship.* Vol. 1, *Report.* Washington, D.C., U.S. Government Printing Office, 1982.

3. Katz J: *The Silent World of Doctor and Patient.* New York, Free Press, 1984.

INDEX

271

and health-care professionals, 3–12,
15–16, 23, 26, 56, 130
health-oriented critique of, 136–141,
144
importance of, 27, 28, 37–41, 57
and incompetency, 59–60, 66, 98, 135
and intentional torts, 114, 116, 118
interactional critique of, 141–143
introduction to, 3–16
and the Judeo-Christian tradition, 17
lack of, 115–118, 123
and the law, 3, 4, 10–14, 35–51, 53–62,
70, 112
literature on, 3–4
and misrepresentation, 177
and negligence, 116–118, 132, 135, 178
noncompliance with, by physicians,
66–67
obtaining, 89, 90, 190, 202
opponents of, 138–141
origin of the term, 39, 131
overall value of, 144–146
and patients, 35–41, 43–49, 53–55, 58,
66, 72–75, 77–78, 115–118, 131–134,
139–140, 155, 160–162, 164–168
and physicians, 3–12, 28, 31, 35–38,
70–71, 102, 112–113, 119, 132, 145,
152, 153, 155, 169, 202–204
and physicians in control of, 140–141,
161
presumption of, 177
problems regarding, 242–249
proponents of, 136–137
purposes of, 241–242, 246, 250
a reasonable approach to, 4, 31, 242–
258
and redress by patients in court, 10,
13–15, 35–43, 112–129. *See also*
Rules for recovery
and refusal to give, 11, 57, 70, 92, 115,
126, 191
requirement of, 57–62, 67, 112, 126,
202–204
to research, 211–219, 224–225, 238
and selection of a course of medical
care, 3, 8–9, 26, 70–71
and self-determination in medical

decisions, 3, 8–9, 26, 44, 59, 66–67,
70–72, 77, 89, 132, 136
and signing of a consent form, 8, 126,
169, 175, 180, 185–187, 225
skepticism about, 140, 141
and societal values, 67, 193
in a specific case, 5–8, 36–39
synthetic approach to, 143–146
terminology of, 12–16
and the therapeutic misconception,
249–258
and therapeutic privilege, 66, 72–78
tighter requirements for, 137
and tort law, 114
and understanding, 57–60, 135, 138–
140, 143, 144, 183, 187–188
and utilitarianism, 23
and voluntariness, 57, 60–62, 71–72
and waiver, 66, 69–72, 186
Informed consent in practice, 151–174.
See also Informed consent
event model of, 151–156
process model of, 151, 156–158
stages of treatment in the process
model, 158–173
Ingelfinger, Franz, 138, 139, 243
Injury-causation, 119–122
Institutional review boards (IRBs), 218
and deception research, 225–226
and disclosure, 224–225
and exempt research, 222–223
and expedited review of research, 223–
224
role of, 220–222, 226, 228–230, 244,
250, 255
shortcomings of, 227–228
variation among, 227–228
and waiver, 225
Instruction directives, by surrogates, 97–
98
Integrity
definition of, 13
legal right of, 13, 35–36, 59, 126, 263
in research, 237
Intentional tort, 114, 116, 118
Interactionist critique, 141–143
Intoxication, and incompetency, 87–89

and ethics and consent and
relationship with patients, 3–16, 26,
28, 35, 52–54, 59–62, 112, 116, 124,
126, 132, 139–140, 145, 151–173,
175–183, 185–188, 194–204, 265, 269
and goals, 219, 237–238
and incompetency, 84–87, 89–94, 96,
101–106, 108, 109, 200–201
and judicial review, 102–103, 109
legal rule for, regarding patients'
consent, 36–37, 66–67, 114–116,
125–126, 146
and liability, 103–105, 108, 109, 114,
176, 177
and litigation, 113, 117, 119–122, 124–
127
and negligence, 115–121, 126
noncompliance by, regarding informed
consent, 67
opposition of, to informed consent,
131–136, 138–146, 202, 264
and options, 53–54
and patients in research, 216
penalties for, 3, 14–16, 134, 137, 143–
144
reeducation of, 133, 145–146, 264–269
and refusal of treatment by patients,
194–204
and risks, 50–54, 268
and rules for recovery, 31
and surrogates, 103–104, 108
and therapeutic privilege, 72–78
and waiver, 70–72
Placebo, 239, 243, 246, 251, 252
Pluralistic deontology, 22 n.
Podiatrists, and informed consent, 15
Police power
and governmental protection of health,
29
and vaccination, 29
President's Commission for the Study of
Ethical Problems in Medicine and
Biomedical and Behavioral
Research, 12, 137, 163, 263
Presumptions in law, 177–179
Preventive medicine, 28, 203
Privacy, law of, 36, 166

Procedure
alternative to a medical, 54–55
nature of a medical, 50
Process model of informed consent, 151,
156
advantages of, 157–158
ascertaining the goals of treatment,
158, 162–164
defining the problem, 158, 160–162
disadvantages of, 158
establishing the relationship, 158–160
follow-up, 158, 169–172
importance of joint patient-physician
decision making in, 158
and legal requirements, 157
mutual monitoring, 156–157
selecting a therapeutic plan, 158, 164–
169
stages of treatment in the, 158–173
Professional medical ethics, 105
Professional standards of disclosure, 41–
45, 48, 131, 134
Protestant theology, and the individual
conscience, 26
Proxy, and incompetency, 94, 95, 97
Psychiatric patients, and right of refusal,
193–194, 198
Psychiatrists, and rejection of treatment,
200
Psychic integrity. *See* Integrity
Psychologists, and informed consent, 15
Psychoses, and incompetency, 87–88,
101, 198
Public Health Service, policy of, on
research programs, 217
Public involvement, in informed consent,
27

Quarantine laws, 29
Quinlan case (1976), 106, 107, 191

Ramsey, P., 241, 257
Randomization
and decision making, 240, 241
ethics of, 239, 240
to minimize bias, 238, 240
problems of, 243, 245